PDR CLINICAL HANDBOOK:

Hyperlipidemia

SCOTT M. GRUNDY, *M.D., Ph.D.*
Director, Center for Human Nutrition
Distinguished Professor of Internal Medicine
Chairman, Department of Clinical Nutrition
University of Texas Southwestern Medical Center
Dallas, Texas

PDR CLINICAL HANDBOOK: HYPERLIPIDEMIA

SCOTT M. GRUNDY, MD, PhD
Director, Center for Human Nutrition
Distinguished Professor of Internal Medicine
Chairman, Department of Clinical Nutrition
University of Texas SW Medical Center, Dallas, Texas

Editor: Edward P. Connor
Art Director: Robert Hartman
Manager of Production Operations: Thomas Westburgh
Project Manager: Lynn S. Wilhelm
Production Design Supervisor: Adeline Rich
Electronic Publishing Designers: Bryan Dix, Rosalia Sberna, Livio Udina

PHYSICIANS' DESK REFERENCE

Executive Vice President, Directory Services: Paul Walsh
Vice President, Clinical Communications and
   Strategic Initiatives: Mukesh Mehta, RPh
Vice President, Sales and Marketing: Dikran N. Barsamian
Director of Trade Sales: Bill Gaffney
Director of Product Management: Valerie Berger
Senior Product Manager: Jeffrey D. Dubin
Senior Director, Operations: Brian Holland
Senior Director, Publishing Sales and Marketing: Michael Bennett
Direct Mail Managers: Jennifer M. Fronzaglia, Lorraine M. Loening
Promotion Manager: Linda Levine

ISBN: 1-56363-456-2

HYPERLIPIDEMIA:

Table of Contents

TABLES

Introduction

The National Cholesterol Education Program (NCEP) recently released the third report of the Expert Panel on Detection, Evaluation and Treatment of High Blood Cholesterol in Adults [Adult Treatment Panel III (ATP III)].[1] This report offers clinical guidelines for cholesterol management by health professionals. They complement the NCEP's public health recommendations for reducing risk for coronary heart disease (CHD) through population-based approaches for lowering serum cholesterol. In fact, as more people gain access to programs of disease prevention, public health recommendations and clinical guidelines are becoming increasingly intertwined.

ATP reports are the product of a panel of experts who are appointed by the National Heart, Lung and Blood Institute (NHLBI), which sponsors the NCEP. ATP III was commissioned by the Coordinating Committee of the NCEP. The Coordinating Committee is composed of 41 members who represent many of the major health-professional organizations of the United States. The development of ATP III took 18 months, and several drafts of the report were reviewed by the Coordinating Committee members and the organizations they represent, by another body of experts chosen by NHLBI, and by experts within NHLBI. This extensive review helped to ensure a broad-based and unbiased report.

The ATP III panel was under a mandate from NHLBI and the NCEP Coordinating Committee to produce an evidence-based report. ATP III aims to provide guidelines that afford maximal benefit to patients at acceptable cost-effectiveness of therapy. The panel thus extensively reviewed the existing literature, which served as the foundation for the report. Evidence was classified according to type and strength. Particular emphasis was placed on results of controlled clinical trials for making treatment recommendations. However, other types of data—epidemiological, metabolic studies, and clinical observation—contributed to refinement of recommendations. A group of evidence statements was developed, and these served as the foundation for treatment recommendations.

The ATP III project has resulted in several products. The Executive Summary was published in the *Journal of the American Medical Association (JAMA)* on May 16, 2001.[1] This summary provides details for clinical management of patients with cholesterol disorders. The Full Report will be published by the U.S. Government Printing Office, and likely will be published in a major medical journal as well. The Full Report provides the evidence base for the Executive Summary. It also contains references to the literature that provide the rationale outlined in the present review; this review therefore will not be extensively referenced. The full ATP III provides extensive reference materials for development of new programs for clinical implementation. All of the ATP III products are available on the NHLBI website (www.nhlbi.nih.gov). Besides the Executive Summary and Full Report, the website contains a Palm Pilot tool for application of the guidelines, a quick desk reference of Guidelines At-A-Glance, and patient materials.

ATP III is meant to be a guide to clinical management of patients at risk for CHD and who have cholesterol disorders. It is not intended to be a "standard of care." Scientific evidence developed through clinical trials and other types of research sheds light on general questions. Clinical practice in contrast deals with specific patients who typically present a unique set of problems. Clinical judgment therefore must always be the final arbiter for decisions of clinical management.

Major Features of ATP Reports

ADULT TREATMENT PANEL REPORT I (ATP I)

The NCEP was commissioned by NHLBI in 1985; then in 1988, the first clinical guideline (ATP I) was issued.[2] The major emphasis of ATP I was on primary prevention—the prevention of new onset CHD. Less attention was given to secondary prevention, i.e., cholesterol-lowering therapy in patients with established CHD. The recommendations of ATP I rested largely on the epidemiological association between serum cholesterol levels and CHD incidence. However, the decisions to start NCEP and to produce ATP I were strongly influenced by the Lipid Research Clinics Coronary Primary Prevention Trial (LRC-CPPT).[3] This trial showed that cholesterol lowering with cholestyramine therapy in patients with hyper-cholesterolemia will reduce risk for CHD. Of great importance, ATP I identified elevated LDL cholesterol as the primary target of therapy. It proposed that first-line therapy for treatment of hypercholesterolemia be dietary therapy. Drug therapy was largely reserved for patients who have persistently high LDL-cholesterol levels.

ADULT TREATMENT PANEL REPORT II (ATP II)

Cholesterol guidelines were updated as ATP II in 1993.[4] ATP II endorsed the previous recommendation of treatment of elevated LDL cholesterol for primary prevention; at the same time it added a new emphasis, namely, more intensive LDL-lowering therapy in patients with established CHD (secondary prevention). This new emphasis was based on the meta-analysis of earlier secondary prevention clinical trials that showed a definite benefit from lowering cholesterol levels in patients with established CHD.[4] In ATP II, the goal for LDL cholesterol for CHD patients was set at ≤100 mg/dL. The scientific basis for this goal was derived from multiple lines of evidence, especially meta-analysis of clinical trials and prospective epidemiological evidence.[5]

ADULT TREATMENT PANEL REPORT III (ATP III)

The current ATP III report endorses the recommendations of ATP II, but goes further in intensifying LDL-lowering therapy for several subgroups of the population. This intensification of therapy is made possible by reports of several major clinical trials that were published after 1993. These trials showed a broad benefit in CHD risk reduction resulting from intensive LDL-lowering therapy. The trials were made possible in large part by the advent of HMG CoA reductase inhibitors (statins), which are powerful drugs for reducing serum LDL cholesterol. These major trials,[6] as well as several smaller trials of statin therapy[7] provide a strong evidence base for the new recommendations.

A major new emphasis of ATP III is intensification of management of persons at higher risk who do not yet have established CHD. Thus, ATP III gives a renewed emphasis to primary prevention. However, in contrast to ATP I, which focused almost exclusively on patients with high LDL, ATP III stresses the benefits of cholesterol-lowering therapy in persons at higher risk for CHD regardless of LDL levels. All persons who were candidates for clinical management in ATP I and II still receive clinical attention in ATP III; but ATP III recommends more intensive cholesterol management for persons deemed to be at higher risk for CHD even when serum cholesterol levels are not definitely elevated. This fundamental shift in perspective allows for a substantial expansion of cholesterol-lowering therapy, particularly for use of cholesterol-lowering drugs.

Relation of Serum Cholesterol to Coronary Heart Disease

SERUM CHOLESTEROL AND LIPOPROTEINS

Cholesterol is a vital substance contributing to cell membrane structure besides being a source for steroid hormones and bile acids. Because of its insolubility in water cholesterol must be solubilized in serum by other lipids and specialized proteins that combine to form particles called lipoproteins. Three major classes of lipoproteins carry cholesterol—triglyceride-rich lipoproteins (TGRLP), LDL, and high density lipoproteins (HDL). Cholesterol enters the circulation from either the gut or liver associated with TGRLP. Gut-derived TGRLP contain newly absorbed fat and are called chylomicrons, whereas liver-derived TGRLP are named very low density lipoproteins (VLDL). As TGRLP lose their triglyceride through lipolysis, residual particles called lipoprotein remnants are produced. Chylomicron remnants are removed directly by the liver. VLDL remnants are partly removed by the liver, but also are converted to LDL. Both VLDL remnants and LDL are enriched in cholesterol. LDL likewise returns to the liver, but also can deliver cholesterol to various tissues of the body. In contrast, HDL plays a role in reverse cholesterol transport, i.e., it can return tissue cholesterol to the liver.

When circulating lipoproteins filter into the intima of arteries, they can serve as inflammatory agents to initiate atherogenesis. Different lipoproteins carry different atherogenic potentials and are discussed in the following sections.

LDL CHOLESTEROL AND ATHEROGENESIS

All ATP reports have identified LDL as the major atherogenic lipoprotein. This cholesterol-enriched particle readily filters into the intima of the arterial wall. There it has several adverse actions.[8] It can be first modified by aggregation, oxidation, or chemical modification; then these LDL products become chemoattractants that draw monocytes into the subendothelial space. Tissue macrophages derived from circulating monocytes are the hallmark of early atherosclerotic lesions. These cells engulf modified LDL and become cholesterol-enriched foam cells. Activated macrophages produce cytokines that initiate other steps in atherogenesis, e.g., invasion of smooth muscle cells and deposition of fibrous tissue. Excess LDL alone can induce full-blown atherosclerosis with CHD, as shown in children and adolescents who have severe forms of hypercholesterolemia.

An important concept that has emerged is that LDL is a proinflammatory factor. It is well recognized that atherogenesis is an inflammatory process. In the past, it was believed that lipid accumulation and inflammation proceeded in parallel but somewhat independently. However, a unifying concept is that LDL itself is proinflammatory. This concept has been supported recently by studies which show that lowering of LDL and other lipids causes a lowering of serum C-reactive protein (CRP), an indicator of an ongoing state of inflammation.[9]

Multiple lines of evidence show that elevated LDL cholesterol contributes importantly to development of CHD. This evidence includes studies in experimental animals, epidemiological data, genetic forms of hypercholesterolemia, cellular studies, and controlled clinical trials. The reduction of CHD risk observed in controlled clinical trials of LDL-lowering therapy provides perhaps the strongest evidence for atherogenic potential for elevated LDL cholesterol.[6] These trials include both primary and secondary trials. A meta-analysis of these trials shows benefit from all modalities of LDL lowering (Figure 1).[10] Since 1993, six major trials with statin therapy have been reported. These major clinical trials were:

- Scandinavian Simvastatin Survival Study (4S)[11]
- Cholesterol and Recurrent Events (CARE)[12]
- Long-Term Intervention with Pravastatin in Ischaemic Disease (LIPID)[13]
- West of Scotland Coronary Prevention Study (WOSCOPS)[14]
- Air Force/Texas Coronary Atherosclerosis Prevention Study (AFCAPS/TexCAPS)[15]
- Heart Protection Study (HPS)[16]

In aggregate, these trials reveal that intensive lowering of LDL cholesterol reduces risk for major coronary events (unstable angina, myocardial infarction, coronary death), coronary artery procedures (angioplasty and coronary bypass surgery), stroke, and total mortality (Figure 2). They also demonstrate that LDL-lowering therapy is effective in all categories of patients: those with and without established CHD; men and women, middle-aged and older persons; patients with and without diabetes, and those with and without other risk factors (i.e., cigarette smoking, hypertension) (Figure 3); they also reduce risk regardless of the lipid and lipoprotein profile (Figure 4).

In addition, a series of smaller studies have been reported involving statin therapy that show benefit for reducing progression or enhancing regression of coronary lesions (Figure 5);[7] these trials further reveal significant reduction of major coronary events in patients treated with statin therapy over the relatively short period of LDL-lowering drug therapy (Figure 6).[7]

Besides clinical trials, many prospective studies call attention to the fact that serum LDL-cholesterol levels (often shown by serum total cholesterol levels) are predictive of CHD risk over a broad range of LDL-cholesterol levels. On the basis of many studies, the general relation between LDL cholesterol and CHD is now known. As LDL-cholesterol levels rise, risk for CHD increases exponentially (or log-linearly).[17] In population, absolute risk for CHD is low when LDL-cholesterol levels are <100 mg/dL, even when other risk factors are present. Hence an LDL-cholesterol level <100 mg/dL can be called optimal.

Based on these multiple lines of evidence, ATP III proposes the following classification for

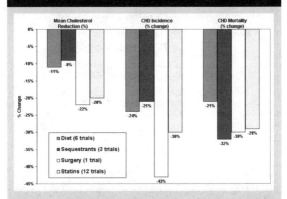

Figure 1 - Coronary Heart Disease (CHD) outcomes in clinical trials of cholesterol-lowering therapy (modified from ATP III). Meta-analysis of clinical trials with diet (6 trials), bile acid sequestrants (3 trials), surgery (ileal exclusion operation) (1 trial), and statins (12 trials).

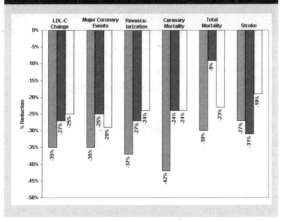

Figure 2 - LDL-Cholesterol (LDL-C), cardiovascular outcomes, and total mortality outcome in clinical trials with statins (modified from ATP III meta-analysis).

Figure 3 - Risk reductions for major coronary events (hard CHD) in various subgroups of major statin trials (modified from ATP III meta-analysis). Statin therapy produced significant reductions in risk for CHD in all subgroups.

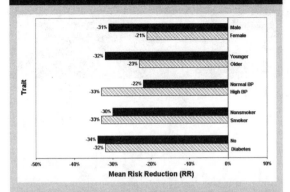

Figure 4 - Risk reductions for major coronary events (hard CHD) according to lipid and lipoprotein levels in major statin trials (modified from ATP III meta-analysis). Statin therapy reduced risk for CHD in all subgroups. Abbreviations: TC = Total Cholesterol; LDL-C = LDL Cholesterol; HDL-C = HDL Cholesterol; TG = Triglyceride.

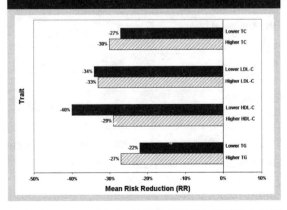

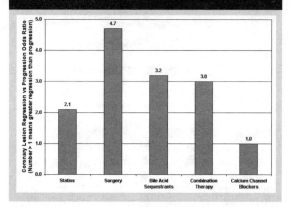

Figure 5—Odds ratio for coronary lesions regression vs. progression in angiographic trials of LDL lowering therapy (modified from ATP III meta-analysis). Numbers greater than 1.0 denote greater regression than progression of coronary lesions. All LDL-lowering therapies produced more regression than progression. In contrast, calcium channel blockers did not produce significant changes, whereas placebo therapy led to more progression than regression. Surgery represents the ileal exclusion operation.

LDL cholesterol:

LDL Cholesterol Level	Category
<100 mg/dL	Optimal
100-129 mg/dL	Near optimal/above optimal
130-159 mg/dL	Borderline high
160-189 mg/dL	High
≥190 mg/dL	Very high

A large body of evidence indicates that elevated concentrations of LDL contribute to coronary atherosclerosis and development of CHD throughout

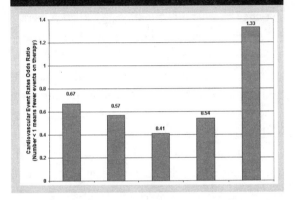

Figure 6–Ratios of cardiovascular events in angiographic trials of LDL-lowering therapies (modified from ATP III meta-analysis). Ratios less than 1.0 signify fewer events with LDL-lowering therapy than with placebo over the duration of the study. Surgery represents the ileal exclusion operation.

the pathogenic process. For instance, higher levels of LDL initiate atherogenesis and promote the formation of atherosclerotic plaques.[18] The rate of formation of plaques is accentuated when other CHD risk factors are present. Atherosclerotic lesions first appear in adolescence as "fatty streaks" and then into middle age are gradually transformed into "fibrous plaques." Although fibrous plaques may partially occlude the arterial lumen, they tend to be stable lesions because a thick fibrous cap protects them against rupture. When such plaques grow large enough they can lead to angina pectoris. Anginal chest pain commonly develops when the lumen of the coronary artery is 50-70% obstructed. As fibrous plaques enlarge some of these become "unstable" and are vulnerable to rupture. Unstable plaques typically have a thin fibrous cap covering an underlying area of macrophage-enriched chronic inflammation.[19] When vulnerable plaques rupture, loss of the endothelial covering exposes a highly thrombogenic surface that elicits an overlying thrombosis. Plaque rupture and consequent thrombus formation account for most acute coronary syndromes (unstable angina and myocardial infarction).[20] High levels of circulating LDL contribute to all forms of atherosclerosis. LDL is a proinflammatory agent that initiates and sustains every stage of atherogenesis. In fact, elevated serum LDL can be considered the primary atherogenic factor because when LDL levels in populations are very low, CHD is relatively rare, even when other risk factors are common.

TRIGLYCERIDE-RICH LIPOPROTEINS, VLDL CHOLESTEROL, AND ATHEROGENESIS

Several types of TGRLP occur in the circulation, and their atherogenic potentials appear to differ. Native chylomicrons probably do not produce atherosclerosis; however cholesterol-enriched chylomicron remnants likely can promote atherogenesis. Similarly, newly secreted VLDL may not be directly atherogenic, whereas cholesterol-enriched VLDL remnants almost certainly are. ATP III thus identified VLDL cholesterol, which is a surrogate marker for VLDL remnants, as one form of "atherogenic cholesterol." In patients with elevated triglycerides, VLDL-cholesterol levels can be considerably increased and thereby can contribute substantially to atherogenesis. ATP III thus recognizes a high VLDL cholesterol as a potential target of cholesterol-lowering therapy in addition to elevated LDL cholesterol.

Because of the atherogenic potential of VLDL cholesterol, ATP III identifies the combination of LDL cholesterol + VLDL cholesterol as a secondary target of treatment after LDL. This combination of two atherogenic forms of cholesterol is called non-HDL cholesterol; it includes all cholesterol in serum except for that in HDL cholesterol. Normally, non-HDL cholesterol is about 30 mg/dL higher than is LDL cholesterol. Consequently non-HDL cholesterol as a secondary target of treatment has a goal of therapy 30 mg/dL higher than the goal for LDL cholesterol.

An elevated TGRLP is associated with increased risk for CHD in ways that go beyond the atherogenic potential of cholesterol-enriched TGRLP. Raised triglycerides often signify the presence of other metabolic risk factors that contribute to atherogenesis and to acute coronary syndromes. This constellation of risk factors is discussed in more detail under the section on the Metabolic Syndrome, for which an elevated triglyceride is a common marker.

ATP III provides a new classification for serum triglycerides that takes into account both the atherogenic potential of cholesterol-enriched TGRLP and the association of elevated triglyceride with the metabolic syndrome. This classification is as follows:

Triglyceride Level	Category
150-199 mg/dL	Borderline high
200-499 mg/dL	High
≥500 mg/dL	Very high

LOW HDL CHOLESTEROL AS A RISK FACTOR

Epidemiological studies reveal that low levels of serum HDL cholesterol associate with increased risk for CHD. The mechanisms underlying this association remain to be fully elucidated. Some evidence suggests that HDL plays a role in reverse cholesterol transport, i.e., in removal of excess cholesterol from tissues for transport to the liver. One site of this excess cholesterol could be the arterial wall plaque. Other protective actions of HDL have been postulated, e.g., prevention of LDL aggregation and oxidation and transport of other arterial protective substances. Equally important appears to be the fact that low HDL-cholesterol concentrations often point to other metabolic risk factors characteristic of the metabolic syndrome. This latter connection frequently occurs with only moderate reductions in HDL cholesterol. Especially for this latter reason, ATP III set a higher concentration to define a low HDL-cholesterol level (<40 mg/dL) than was used in ATP I and II, the latter being <35 mg/dL.

ATHEROGENIC DYSLIPIDEMIA: THE ATHEROGENIC LIPID TRIAD

A trio of lipoprotein abnormalities is called atherogenic dyslipidemia. It consists of the following changes:

- Elevated serum triglyceride (≥150 mg/dL)

- Small LDL particles

- Reduced HDL cholesterol
  [<40 mg/dL (men); <50 mg/dL (women)]

Atherogenic dyslipidemia commonly is present in persons with premature CHD. It appears to partner with elevated LDL cholesterol to promote development of atherosclerosis. It commonly occurs in persons who are overweight/ obese and are physically inactive. In some people, however, one or another of the components of this lipid triad are accentuated by genetic factors.

NON-HDL CHOLESTEROL AND APOLIPOPROTEIN B

There is increasing evidence that most lipoproteins that contain apolipoprotein B (apo B) are atherogenic. Although the atherogenic potential of different apo B-containing lipoproteins may vary, total apo B levels correlate positively with risk for CHD. Some investigators have proposed that measurement of total apo B might be preferred to LDL cholesterol in the prediction of CHD risk. ATP III however did not recommend routine measurement of apo B for the following reasons: (a) epidemiological studies that show superiority of prediction for total apo B over LDL cholesterol are limited, (b) several methodological issues for accurate and routine measurement of total apo B remain unresolved, and (c) measurements of total apo B in clinical laboratories are not routinely available. However, ATP III did recognize a need to include the cholesterol of remnant lipoproteins along with LDL cholesterol as a target of therapy in patients with elevated triglycerides. For this reason, non-HDL cholesterol was identified as a secondary target of cholesterol-lowering therapy in patients with high triglycerides (≥200 mg/dL). Non-HDL cholesterol is calculated as total cholesterol − HDL cholesterol, and it includes LDL cholesterol + VLDL cholesterol. Furthermore, non-HDL cholesterol is highly correlated with total apo B. Thus, for most persons, measurement of non-HDL cholesterol obviates the need for determination of total apo B.

Risk Evaluation: Critical Component of ATP III

The new emphasis of ATP III on high-risk primary prevention requires more attention to determination of risk status. CHD is a multifactorial disease, and the likelihood for its occurrence depends on the identification of the many factors responsible for atherogenesis. To fully understand the rationale for the new guidelines for high-risk primary prevention one must appreciate the issues associated with risk assessment. The following provides a summary of the key issues.

ABSOLUTE RISK VS. RELATIVE RISK

Earlier epidemiological studies stressed the relative contribution of individual risk factors to total CHD risk. More recently emphasis has shifted to absolute risk, i.e., the likelihood for developing CHD in a given amount of time. Absolute risk

estimations require an assessment of all factors
known to affect risk. For this reason, absolute
risk projection is sometimes called global risk
assessment; this term implies that all risk factors
are combined to form a single risk projection.
ATP III supports measurement of absolute risk as
the essential aim of risk assessment.

As shown in Table 1, ATP III specifies three
categories of absolute risk: high risk, intermediate risk, and lower risk. High risk subdivides
into established CHD and CHD risk equivalents.
Patients with established CHD are at high risk
for suffering major coronary events (myocardial
infarction and coronary death in the near
future); those with CHD risk equivalents do not
have evident CHD but they carry as high an

Table 1–Absolute Risk Categories

- High risk
  - Coronary heart disease (CHD)
  - CHD risk equivalents
- Intermediate risk
  - Moderately high risk
  - Moderate risk
- Lower risk

---

absolute risk for future major coronary events as
do patients with established CHD. The interme-

diate-risk category includes patients at moderately high or moderate risk. Finally, many people in the general population are at relatively low-absolute risk.

SHORT-TERM VS. LONG-TERM RISK

ATP III defines a high risk in the short term as a high likelihood of developing a major coronary event (myocardial infarction and coronary death) sometime in the next decade (Table 2). Many persons who have a high short-term risk carry unstable coronary plaques that are prone to rupture; when this occurs, a major coronary event follows. Consequently the goal of short-term risk reduction is to prevent plaque rupture and hence major coronary events (Table 2). A high long-term risk signifies a high likelihood of experiencing CHD sometime over a lifetime. A person at high long-term risk presumably is developing coronary atherosclerosis at an increased rate although plaques presumably will not grow enough to become unstable plaques earlier in life; therefore, these persons will not have a high short-term risk. It thus follows that the goal of therapy in such persons is to prevent de novo development of coronary atherosclerosis and thus to reduce the lifetime risk for CHD.

Table 2–Short-Term vs. Long-Term Risk

• High short-term risk (≤10 years)
  - Pathogenesis: formation of unstable coronary plaques in pre-existing atherosclerotic lesions
  - Goal of preventive therapy: to stabilize coronary plaques thereby preventing major coronary events (unstable angina and myocardial infarction)

• High long-term risk (>10 years)
  - Pathogenesis: De novo development of coronary atherosclerosis
  - Goal of preventive therapy: to prevent de novo development of coronary atherosclerosis so as to reduce risk for CHD over a lifetime

---

Because of the introduction of safe and effective drugs to rapidly reduce risk for CHD, more attention has been given to short-term projections of risk (e.g., ≤10 years). Patients found to be at high risk in the short term are often candidates for LDL-lowering drugs and other risk-reducing agents (e.g., antihypertensive drugs or low-dose aspirin). The goal of intensive therapy in the short term is to prevent coronary plaque rupture and acute coronary syndromes. It is assumed that most persons at high short-term risk already have advanced coronary atherosclerosis; for this reason, priority is given to prevention of plaque rupture and acute coronary syndromes. ATP III has uncovered a greater number of persons at high short-term risk who are candidates for LDL-lowering drugs than were identified in previous ATP reports.

Nevertheless, ATP III by no means ignores long-term lifetime risk. Persons at high lifetime risk deserve attention in clinical management even when they are not at high risk in the short term. The goal of long-term risk reduction is to prevent the development of atherosclerosis in the first place. To reduce the burden of atherosclerotic disease in our society, a greater effort must be given to preventing earlier stages of atherosclerosis. Most persons at high long-term risk will be candidates for therapeutic lifestyle changes to reduce risk. Nevertheless those with very high LDL cholesterol or high LDL cholesterol plus other risk factors may well benefit from cholesterol-lowering drugs even when short-term risk is not high. One principle of risk management is that every categorical risk factor deserves clinical management, whether it be cigarette smoking, hypertension, diabetes, or hypercholesterolemia. This principle should not be overlooked even though priority goes to short-term risk assessment.

CHD AS AN ABSOLUTE RISK INDICATOR

By ATP III convention, the following conditions constitute a diagnosis of CHD.

- History of myocardial infarction
- History of unstable or stable angina pectoris
- History of coronary artery procedures (angioplasty or coronary artery surgery)
- Evidence of ischemic heart disease by stress testing

Once a person has clinically manifest CHD this person is at high risk for future major coronary events. Most persons with clinical CHD already have advanced coronary atherosclerosis and are at increased likelihood for suffering yet another plaque rupture causing an acute coronary syndrome. In the past, 10-year risk for serious CHD events (myocardial infarction or coronary death) approached 50%. The events are called *hard* CHD. However, because of advances in medical management, the 10-year risk for hard CHD in persons with previous myocardial infarction has fallen to about 25%. This risk level is revealed from CHD rates in the placebo groups of secondary prevention trials of statin therapy.[12,13] Moreover, other studies show that

persons with stable angina have a 10-year risk
for hard CHD events of about 20%. All of these
percentages are in the absence of LDL-lowering
drugs. The value of >20% per decade for hard
CHD (myocardial infarction and coronary death)
thus sets a standard by which to evaluate the
absolute risk status of patients without CHD.

CONCEPT OF CHD RISK EQUIVALENTS

The concept of CHD risk equivalents is one of
the most important innovations of ATP III.
According to this concept, some persons without
clinically manifest CHD have as high a risk for
hard CHD events as do those with established
CHD. Such persons are said to have a *CHD
risk equivalent.* It follows from this concept
that persons with CHD risk equivalents warrant
the same intensity of risk reduction therapy as
do patients with established CHD. ATP III doc-
uments three conditions that convey a CHD risk
equivalent: these are (a) non-coronary forms of
clinical atherosclerotic disease, (b) diabetes, and
(c) multiple-risk factors that raise 10-year risk
for hard CHD to be above 20%.

CLINICAL CATEGORIES OF CHD RISK EQUIVALENTS

Non-Coronary Forms of Atherosclerotic Disease
Atherosclerosis tends to be generalized; athero-

sclerotic disease in one region of the arterial tree is usually associated with atherosclerosis in other regions. Causation of atherosclerosis seemingly is similar in coronary, peripheral, and carotid arteries. Likewise, clinical atherosclerotic disease in non-coronary arterial beds has independent predictive power for new CHD events. Indeed, certain forms of clinical atherosclerotic disease carry as high a risk for future major coronary events as does established CHD. Based on an extensive review of the literature, ATP III uncovered three forms of clinical atherosclerotic disease that qualify for being CHD risk equivalents.

- Atherosclerotic peripheral arterial disease
- Atherosclerotic abdominal aortic aneurysm
- Symptomatic carotid artery disease (including transient cerebral attacks of carotid origin, carotid stroke, and ≥50% stenosis of carotid arteries)

Diabetes

It should be noted that in ATP I and ATP II diabetes mellitus was listed as a major factor to modify goals for LDL cholesterol in primary prevention. In ATP III however diabetes was re-evaluated and then re-classified as a CHD risk equivalent. Three reasons were specified to justify raising diabetes to a risk category similar to that for patients with established CHD. First, a review of the literature indicated that in high-risk populations most persons with type 2 diabetes have a 10-year risk for hard CHD (myocardial infarction and coronary death) that approximates the risk in CHD patients without diabetes. Second, patients with diabetes at time of acute myocardial infarction have a death rate that is about twice that of non-diabetic persons. And third, patients with diabetes have a relatively poor survival in the long-term after myocardial infarction. The worsened prognosis associated with CHD in persons with diabetes calls for more intensified primary prevention of CHD. For these several reasons, type 2 diabetes is designated a CHD risk equivalent. Persons with type 2 diabetes without CHD therefore should have the same LDL-cholesterol goals as do patients with established CHD.

ATP III also noted that people with type 1 diabetes are at higher risk for CHD. Although some people with type 1 diabetes may not have a 10-year risk for CHD equal to that of CHD patients, they nonetheless are at high long-term risk. ATP III concluded that LDL-lowering therapy would almost certainly reduce the relative risk for CHD similarly in types 1 and 2 diabetes. It therefore was recommended that although clinical judgment be employed whether to use LDL-lowering drugs in patients with type 1 diabetes, as risk begins to rise, LDL-lowering drugs probably are warranted.

Multiple-Risk Factors Causing a High-Risk State

Several risk factors other than diabetes are well established as being independently correlated with development of CHD. In some patients, these risk factors aggregate to the point that a CHD risk equivalent is present. Such patients should benefit similarly from the same intensity of risk reduction that is used in other patients with CHD or other CHD risk equivalents. The identification of these high-risk individuals are examined in more detail in the following section.

MAJOR-RISK FACTORS AS MODIFIERS OF INTENSITY OF PRIMARY PREVENTION

Several risk factors are independently associated with CHD and have a relatively high frequency in the general population. As already discussed, elevated LDL cholesterol is a major risk factor. Risk factors that were specified in ATP III as major risk factors and are used to set goals for LDL-lowering

therapy in primary prevention are the following:
Positive Major-Risk Factors
(other than LDL cholesterol)

- Age (male: ≥45 years; female: ≥55 years)

- Family history of premature CHD (definite myocardial infarction or sudden death before 55 years of age in father or other male first-degree relative, or before 65 years of age in mother or other first-degree relative)

- Current cigarette smoking (any smoking in the past year)

- Hypertension (BP ≥140/90 mmHg, or on anti-hypertensive medication)

- Low HDL cholesterol (<40 mg/dL)

Negative Risk Factor

- High HDL cholesterol (≥60 mg/dL)

The rationale for including each of these risk factors in decisions about LDL-lowering therapy is discussed briefly.

Advancing age is accompanied by a steeply increasing risk for coronary disease in both men and women. The principal reason is that age is a reflection of the progressive accumulation of coronary atherosclerosis. Once atherosclerosis is established, it becomes a risk factor in itself for future major coronary events. Greater accumulations of plaque are accompanied by a greater likelihood of plaque rupture. Since absolute risk for CHD increases more rapidly in men than in women, age counts as a categorical risk factor ten years earlier in men than in women i.e., 45 vs. 55 years of age.

Family history of premature CHD counts as a risk factor to modify LDL goals in ATP III. Many studies support an independent risk predictive power for family history of CHD. Although the Framingham Heart Study did not find enough predictive power to include it in risk scoring, several other reports claim independence of prediction. The ATP III panel therefore concluded that a family history of premature CHD should be added to the list of factors that modify treatment goals for LDL cholesterol.

Cigarette smoking is related to CHD in a dose dependent manner in both men and women. Smoking appears to destabilize coronary plaques and is a particularly strong risk factor for acute coronary syndromes. Conversely, cessation of smoking substantially lowers risk for major coronary events.

Hypertension is a strong risk factor for CHD, stroke, heart failure, and kidney failure. Lowering blood pressure in persons with hypertension will reduce risk for both stroke and major coronary events. Even so, treatment of hypertension does not completely reverse risk for major coronary events associated with the hypertensive state; hence a prior diagnosis of hypertension remains a risk factor even when it is under treatment.

Low HDL cholesterol (<40 mg/dL) counts as a positive risk factor for reasons discussed before. On the other hand, an elevated HDL cholesterol (≥60 mg/dL) denotes a negative risk factor, which allows removal of one positive risk factor in assessment of risk status.

Risk categories based on number of risk factors. ATP III makes a fundamental division of risk categories into (a) multiple (2+) risk factors, and (b) 0-1 risk factors. Persons with multiple (2+) risk factors are a major focus of the new cholesterol guidelines. An important new feature of ATP III is the introduction of Framingham risk scoring to refine estimates of absolute risk in persons with multiple (2+) risk factors. Three different categories receive different intensities of LDL-lowering therapy, depending on the level of risk. They include:

- 10-year risk for CHD >20%
  (CHD risk equivalent)
- 10-year risk for CHD 10-20%
- 10-year risk for CHD <10%

Table 3A–Estimating 10-Year Risk for CHD for Men and Women

Estimate of 10-Year Risk for **Men** (Framingham Point Scores)

Age, y	Points
20-34	-9
35-39	-4
40-44	0
45-49	3
50-54	6
55-59	8
60-64	10
65-69	11
70-74	12
75-79	13

Total Cholesterol, mg/dL	Points				
	Age 20-39 y	Age 40-49 y	Age 50-59 y	Age 60-69 y	Age 70-79 y
<160	0	0	0	0	0
160-199	4	3	2	1	0
200-239	7	5	3	1	0
240-279	9	6	4	2	1
≥280	11	8	5	3	1

	Points				
	Age 20-39 y	Age 40-49 y	Age 50-59 y	Age 60-69 y	Age 70-79 y
Nonsmoker	0	0	0	0	0
Smoker	8	5	3	1	1

HDL, mg/dL	Points
≥60	-1
50-59	0
40-49	1
<40	2

Systolic BP, mm Hg	If Untreated	If Treated
<120	0	0
120-129	0	1
130-139	1	2
140-159	1	2
≥160	2	3

Point Total	10-Year Risk, %
<0	<1
0	1
1	1
2	1
3	1
4	1
5	2
6	2
7	3
8	4
9	5
10	6
11	8
12	10
13	12
14	16
15	20
16	25
≥17	≥30

Table 3B–Estimating 10-Year Risk for CHD for Men and Women *(Continued)*

Estimate of 10-Year Risk for **Women** (Framingham Point Scores)

Age, y	Points
20-34	–7
35-39	–3
40-44	0
45-49	3
50-54	6
55-59	8
60-64	10
65-69	12
70-74	14
75-79	16

Total Cholesterol, mg/dL	Points				
	Age 20-39 y	Age 40-49 y	Age 50-59 y	Age 60-69 y	Age 70-79 y
<160	0	0	0	0	0
160-199	4	3	2	1	1
200-239	8	6	4	2	1
240-279	11	8	5	3	2
≥280	13	10	7	4	2

	Points				
	Age 20-39 y	Age 40-49 y	Age 50-59 y	Age 60-69 y	Age 70-79 y
Nonsmoker	0	0	0	0	0
Smoker	9	7	4	2	1

HDL, mg/dL	Points
≥60	–1
50-59	0
40-49	1
<40	2

Systolic BP, mm Hg	If Untreated	If Treated
<120	0	0
120-129	1	3
130-139	2	4
140-159	3	5
≥160	4	6

Point Total	10-Year Risk, %
<9	<1
9	1
10	1
11	1
12	1
13	2
14	2
15	3
16	4
17	5
18	6
19	8
20	11
21	14
22	17
23	22
24	27
≥25	≥30

A modified Framingham risk algorithm was developed for ATP III (Table 3). This algorithm specifies hard CHD (myocardial infarction and CHD death) as the endpoint of risk assessment. Previously, Framingham algorithms employed total CHD (stable and unstable angina, electro-cardiographic evidence of CHD, myocardial infarction, and coronary death as the endpoint of assessment). Use of hard CHD as the endpoint however allows risk in non-CHD patients to be standardized relative to known risk for major coronary events in patients with established CHD. Furthermore, in 1999, NHLBI sponsored a workshop to compare Framingham predictions for hard CHD with those from other prospective studies in the United States. The results of this comparison revealed that Framingham scoring is transportable to other populations in the United States.[21,22] In other words, the Framingham algorithm for hard CHD provides a valid risk estimate for most populations in the United States. This algorithm can be accessed at the following website:
http://hin.nhlbi.nih.gov/atpiii/calculator.asp

UNDERLYING RISK FACTORS AS DIRECT TARGETS OF INTERVENTION

In addition to the major, independent risk factors that directly promote atherosclerosis,

ATP III recognizes three underlying risk factors that predispose to the major risk factors and may contribute to CHD in other ways. These factors modify a population's underlying (or baseline) risk for CHD. In ATP III they are not used to modify LDL-cholesterol goals, but instead constitute direct targets of therapy. These include:

- Atherogenic diet
- Overweight/obesity
- Physical inactivity

Atherogenic diet: Prospective epidemiological surveys suggest that a large number of dietary factors influence atherogenesis. Some of these, such as dietary saturated fats and cholesterol, directly raise LDL-cholesterol levels and thereby promote atherogenesis through a known mechanism. Moreover, in some countries the habitual diet appears to increase risk for CHD independently of LDL cholesterol, whereas in other countries, the diet appears to protect against CHD. For example, the traditional Mediterranean diet, which is rich in fruits, vegetables, whole grains, fish, olive oil, and moderate amounts of wine, is accompanied by a lower risk for CHD than is the diet in Northern,

Central, and eastern regions of Europe where the incidence of CHD remains high. The Dietary Guidelines for Americans 2000 describes a diet closer in composition to that which is traditionally consumed in the Mediterranean world; both diets appear to be favorable for reducing underlying risk for CHD. ATP III thus recommends the diet composition used in treatment of elevated LDL cholesterol resemble that outlined in Dietary Guidelines for Americans 2000 (http://www.health.gov/dietaryguidelines).

Overweight/Obesity: Approximately 97 million adults in the United States are overweight or obese. Overweight consists of a body mass index (BMI) of 25-29.9 kg/m², whereas obesity is defined as a BMI ≥30 kg/m². Being overweight or obese contributes to CHD, stroke, and all-cause mortality. The effects of these conditions on CHD risk appear to be mediated through dyslipidemia (high LDL cholesterol, low HDL cholesterol, high VLDL and triglyceride), hypertension, and type 2 diabetes. ATP III counts obesity as a major, modifiable risk factor for CHD; nevertheless, the incremental risk imparted by overweight/obesity independently of accompanying risk factors has not been precisely determined. ATP III thus does not count overweight/obesity as risk factors to modify LDL-cholesterol goals in primary prevention. Rather, overweight/obesity should be considered as direct targets of medical intervention to reduce underlying risk. Reducing excess body weight has many benefits unrelated to lowering LDL cholesterol.

Physical inactivity is another major risk factor that underlies occurrence of CHD. Evidence indicates however that some of the increased risk for CHD accompanying physical inactivity can be explained by its effects on the major, independent risk factors. Consequently, a history of physical inactivity was not counted as a risk factor for setting goals for LDL cholesterol in primary prevention; this said, clinical judgment can still be used where appropriate to intensify LDL-lowering therapy in persons who are physically inactive.

Overcoming physical inactivity through regular exercise has favorable effects on various CHD risk factors; it lowers VLDL and triglyceride levels, raises HDL cholesterol, improves insulin sensitivity and may lower blood pressure. For these reasons, regular exercise should be encouraged as part of a risk-reduction regimen. Increased physical activity thus becomes a part of ATP III's therapeutic lifestyle changes for persons entering cholesterol management.

EMERGING RISK FACTORS AS ADJUNCTS FOR RISK PREDICTION IN PRIMARY PREVENTION

Several factors other than major, independent risk factors or underlying risk factors have been found to be associated with a higher risk for CHD. These factors can be called *emerging risk factors*. In general they do not have the multiple lines of evidence required to classify them as major risk factors. Some of the emerging risk factors are potential targets for direct intervention; others may serve as adjuncts to risk prediction to modify LDL management in primary prevention. ATP III reviewed several categories of emerging risk factors including the following:

Emerging Lipid Risk Factors

- Triglycerides
- Lipoprotein remnants
- Lipoprotein (a)
- Small LDL particles
- HDL subspecies ("small HDL particles")
- Apolipoproteins B and AI
- Total cholesterol/HDL cholesterol ratio

Emerging Non-Lipid Risk Factors

- Homocysteine

- Thrombogenic/hemostatic factors
- Inflammatory markers
- Impaired fasting glucose

Subclinical Atherosclerotic Disease

- Ankle-brachial blood pressure index (ABI)
- Tests for myocardial ischemia
- Tests for atherosclerotic plaque burden
  - Carotid intimal medial thickening
  - Coronary calcium

Emerging Lipid Risk Factors. (a) As discussed before, ATP III places increased emphasis on TGRLP and their remnants as atherogenic factors. The approach to their management is presented in detail in ATP III. (b) Lipoprotein (a) levels have been correlated with CHD incidence in several studies, but not in all. ATP III did not recommend routine measurement of Lp (a) for risk assessment, but its measurement was considered an option in selected patients, e.g., those with a strong family history of CHD or familial hypercholesterolemia. (c) Small LDL particles are commonly found in patients with premature CHD; these particles generally accompany elevated triglycerides and low HDL-cholesterol levels. Measurement of small LDL particles is not recommended for routine risk assessment; nevertheless, detection of these particles is a diagnostic option for the identification of atherogenic dyslipidemia. (d) Small HDL species often accompany small LDL and also are correlated with elevated triglycerides and low HDL cholesterol. They too suggest the presence of atherogenic dyslipidemia. (e) Apolipoprotein B levels correlate highly with non-HDL cholesterol; consequently the latter is an adequate marker for apolipoprotein B in most patients. (f) Apolipoprotein AI levels appear to carry little if any extra predictive power beyond that provided by HDL cholesterol. (g) The total cholesterol/ HDL cholesterol ratio is widely employed in risk assessment; however, in ATP III, primary emphasis is placed on individual lipoproteins, namely, LDL cholesterol and VLDL cholesterol. This ratio is not included in routine risk assessment.

Emerging Non-lipid Risk Factors. Several non-lipid factors are included among emerging risk factors. (a) Many reports assert that elevated homocysteine carries independent predictive power. Homocysteine measurement thus is optional, but clinical elevations are not common enough to justify a recommendation of routine measurement. If homocysteine is elevated, administration of folic acid (1 milligram per day) may cause a fall in serum levels. Whether this reduction in homocysteine levels will lower risk for CHD is uncertain. (b) Thrombogenic/ hemostatic factors (e.g., elevated fibrinogen and PAI-1) have been reported to carry predictive power in prospective studies. However, accurate measurements are not routinely available for clinical practice. Moreover, fibrinogen levels tend to be highly variable from day-to-day in individuals. Although thrombogenic factors are predictive of CHD in prospective epidemiological studies, their utility for risk assessment for individuals is uncertain. (c) Inflammatory markers have received increased attention in recent years. They are promising as risk predictors. High-sensitivity C-reactive protein (hs-CRP) is the most readily available measure for an inflammatory marker. Levels above the 75th percentile of a reference population can be taken as a categorical elevation. Levels of hs-CRP that constitute a categorical elevation are in the range >4-to-5 mg/L. If hs-CRP is elevated on multiple occasions, the physician has the option to raise the risk level of a patient to a higher category. (d) Impaired fasting glucose (IFG) (plasma glucose 110-125 mg/dL) in some studies signifies increased risk for CHD. Since the plasma glucose should be measured routinely in adults, IFG may come to light during routine testing. Its presence denotes an increased risk for type 2 diabetes, besides being indicative of higher CHD risk. It is a common abnormality found in persons with the metabolic syndrome. However, in ATP III, presence of IFG does not directly modify LDL-cholesterol goals.

Subclinical Atherosclerotic Disease. The detection of substantial atherosclerosis in various arterial beds carries an increased risk for future major coronary events. Just how much of this predictive power is independent of that accompanying the major-risk factors remains to be determined. This question is of prime importance for the future of coronary risk assessment. A recent report[23] of a conference sponsored by the American Heart Association has reviewed the status of subclinical atherosclerosis in CHD risk prediction. The major conclusions of this conference were summarized and supported in ATP III. (a) For example, it was noted that an abnormal ankle/brachial index (ABI) predicts risk for future major coronary events similar to that of established CHD; in fact, an abnormal ABI essentially equates with a diagnosis of clinical peripheral vascular disease, i.e., a category of CHD risk equivalent. (b) Many reports claim that myocardial ischemic changes during exercise stress testing independently predict major coronary events in some subgroups of the general population. For example, an abnormal exercise ECG in a middle-aged man with risk factors raises risk to the level of a CHD risk equivalent; on the other hand, an "abnormal" exercise ECG in young adults and middle-aged women carries much less predictive power. Moreover, the value of exercise testing in older persons is uncertain. Stress testing with radionuclide scanning (SPECT) is more sensitive than exercise ECG for detecting myocardial ischemia and carries useful predictive information; on the other hand, SPECT testing is expensive and not often abnormal enough to justify testing for myocardial ischemia for the purpose of routine risk assessment in asymptomatic persons. (c) The finding of intimal-medial thickening of carotid arteries by B-mode ultrasonography independently predicts major coronary events. Although this test is potentially useful for changing the risk category of some persons with risk factors, the methodology has not been standardized adequately in a large number of facilities; consequently, a recommendation for routine testing thus cannot be made at this time. (d) Measurement of coronary calcium by electron beam computed tomography (EBCT) or spiral CT gives a good indication of the extent of coronary atherosclerosis. Several studies in fact reveal that severity of coronary calcium accumulation independently predicts CHD events. At the present time, the expense, lack of availability, and uncertainty about quantitative predictive power preclude a recommendation for measurement of coronary calcium for routine risk assessment. Nonetheless the ATP III panel did point out that measurement of coronary calcium is an option for adjusting a person's risk status, beyond the major risk factors. This approach for risk assessment has been recently reviewed.

METABOLIC SYNDROME AS MULTIPLE, INTERRELATED FACTORS THAT RAISE RISK

The metabolic syndrome consists of a constellation of risk factors occurring in one individual. It is a multifactorial disorder in which the dominant causes are the interplay of overweight/obesity, physical inactivity, and genetic factors. Because of the rising prevalence of overweight/ obesity in the United States, the metabolic syndrome has become increasingly common. Most persons with the metabolic syndrome have a condition called insulin resistance, which is a reduced tissue responsiveness to the usual actions of insulin. The metabolic syndrome goes by other names— insulin resistance syndrome, metabolic syndrome X, and the deadly quartet. Since the metabolic syndrome represents a major new emphasis of ATP III, its clinical aspects will be examined in some detail.

Metabolic risk factors. There are five major risk factors of the metabolic syndrome. They include a combination of major-risk factors and emerging risk factors:

- Atherogenic dyslipidemia
- Raised blood pressure
- Insulin resistance ± elevated plasma glucose
- Prothrombotic state
- Proinflammatory state

Atherogenic dyslipidemia consists of the *lipid triad*—raised triglycerides, small LDL particles, and low HDL cholesterol. Blood pressure need be included only to the "high-normal" range, but often is higher. Insulin resistance is present in most persons with the metabolic syndrome. Some individuals with insulin resistance have impaired fasting glucose or impaired glucose tolerance. Those with categorical hyperglycemia (≥ 126 mg/dL) have the metabolic syndrome, but are also said to have type 2 diabetes. A prothrombotic state typically is not identified clinically, but could be detected by high levels of PAI-1 and/or fibrinogen. A proinflammatory state is best detected by elevations of hs-CRP, although high plasma levels of inflammatory cytokines also are present.

Atherogenicity of metabolic syndrome. Because of the aggregation of multiple-risk factors in one person, it has proven difficult to determine the relative contribution of each risk factor to the pathogenesis of atherosclerosis or to the development of CHD. Nonetheless, there is growing evidence that all of the risk factors are involved one way or another in atherogenesis. This evidence derives from several sources, notably, from studies in laboratory animals and in patients who have defects in risk factors. Thus the metabolic syndrome can be viewed as a *multiplex-risk factor,* i.e., a constellation of risk factors acting in concert to promote atherosclerosis and to predispose to CHD.

Risk factors underlying the metabolic syndrome. This syndrome has a multifactorial etiology. The following factors appear to contribute to the metabolic syndrome:

- Overweight/obesity (especially abdominal obesity)
- Physical inactivity
- Genetic susceptibility
- Hormonal factors

● Dietary factors

● Aging

Overweight/obesity (especially abdominal obesity). Most people who develop the metabolic syndrome are overweight (BMI 25-29.9 kg/m²) or obese (BMI ≥30 kg/m²).[24] The link between excess body fat and metabolic-risk factors is not totally understood. One important link appears to be through an excess of circulation of non-esterified fatty acids (NEFA). These are derived from the lipolysis of adipose tissue triglyceride. Many studies show that high NEFA levels accompany excess body fat. This excess leads to increased influx of NEFA into the muscle and liver. This results in insulin resistance in muscle and high-fat content in the liver. Both changes appear to enhance development of metabolic-risk factors. Beyond NEFA however, excess adipose tissue may produce other factors that enhance the high levels of C-reactive protein found in overweight/obesity persons.[25,26] In a word, overweight/obesity induces a proinflammatory state. In addition, an excess of adipose tissue is accompanied by increased secretion of PAI-1, which can shift hemostasis balance to a pro-thrombotic state.[27,28] All of these links between overweight/obesity and the metabolic syndrome are accentuated in people who have abdominal obesity. Apparently accumulation of fat in the abdomen leads to higher levels of NEFA, cytokines, and PAI-1 than fat accumulation elsewhere. These differences probably account for the unusually strong association between abdominal obesity and the metabolic syndrome.

Physical inactivity. Sedentary life habits also are associated with an increased prevalence of the risk factors of the metabolic syndrome.[29,30] Part of this association likely is related to the contribution of sedentary life habits to development of overweight/obesity. In addition, physical inactivity may shift metabolic balance to a unfavorable state through mechanisms that are independent of body fat content. For example, physical activity modifies the metabolism of skeletal muscle to reduce insulin resistance. Whether this effect on insulin resistance in muscle can account for reported improvements in other metabolic risk factors is not certain. Regardless, there is considerable evidence that increased physical activity will favorably modify the risk factors of the metabolic syndrome.

Genetic susceptibility. To develop the metabolic syndrome, some degree of genetic susceptibility appears to be necessary. Many persons have the other factors contributing to the metabolic syndrome, but do not develop the condition because of genetic protection. On the other hand, other people have a genetic susceptibility and acquire the metabolic syndrome even when other underlying risk factors are only mildly expressed. However, even in people who are genetically susceptible, the syndrome typically does not occur in the complete absence of the other risk factors. Moreover, genetic susceptibility determines which metabolic risk factors are most robustly expressed. The following list shows the metabolic phenotypes that are most common in different ethnic groups that are genetically predisposed to this syndrome.

- Caucasians: atherogenic dyslipidemia > hypertension > diabetes
- African Americans: hypertension > diabetes > dyslipidemia
- Native Americans: diabetes > dyslipidemia >> hypertension
- South Asians: coronary heart disease > diabetes > dyslipidemia > hypertension
- East Asians: diabetes > hypertension
- Turkish populations: low HDL cholesterol

In Caucasians, atherogenic dyslipidemia is common, but with aging, hypertension becomes more predominant. With the increase in obesity and sedentary life habits in North America and

Europe, the incidence of type 2 diabetes is rising; but even so, diabetes is less common than in some populations. The primary manifestation of the metabolic syndrome in African Americans is hypertension;[31] however, increasing obesity has contributed to a rising prevalence of diabetes. In contrast, atherogenic dyslipidemia is less common in African Americans than in Caucasians. Native Americans are predisposed to type 2 diabetes as the primary manifestation of the metabolic syndrome;[32] less common in this population are dyslipidemia and hypertension. South Asians are highly susceptible to the metabolic syndrome, which develops with only mild obesity.[33,34] In this population, coronary heart disease often occurs even without severely abnormal metabolic risk factors.[35] In South Asia, the incidence of diabetes also is unusually high, whereas dyslipidemia and hypertension are not unusually common. In contrast, type 2 diabetes and hypertension appear to be the major manifestations of the metabolic syndrome in East Asians;[36] CHD appears to be less common than diabetes in this population.[37] Finally, the population in Turkey is of interest in that a low serum HDL is genetically frequent, and this abnormality is the primary metabolic risk factor observed in patients with the metabolic syndrome.[38]

Hormonal factors. In middle age, men are more susceptible to the development of the metabolic syndrome. This greater susceptibility has been attributed to the propensity of men to develop abdominal obesity as well as to the action of testosterone to reduce HDL-cholesterol levels. A role for androgens is suggested in women with polycystic ovary syndrome who exhibit hyperandrogenemia and are prone to the metabolic syndrome.[39] All this does not mean that other women are immune to the metabolic syndrome. Women who are obese and physically inactive often exhibit insulin resistance and the metabolic syndrome. In fact, much of premature CHD in women appears to occur in women who have either the metabolic syndrome or type 2 diabetes.

Dietary nutrient composition. Whether the nutrient composition of the diet affects the propensity for the metabolic syndrome has been a matter of dispute. Recently, some investigators have expressed concern that diets high in carbohydrates may predispose to the metabolic syndrome.[40] At present, all that can be said is that high-carbohydrate diets worsen some of the risk factors of this syndrome. For example, high-carbohydrate diets tend to raise serum triglyceride and to lower HDL-cholesterol levels. They also increase postprandial responses to plasma glucose and insulin. Whether prolonged "over stimulation" of insulin secretion by high-carbohydrates diets accelerates the age-related decline in beta-cell release of insulin remains in the area of speculation at present. The effects of high-carbohydrate diets to worsen some metabolic risk factors led the ATP III panel to recommended replacement of some dietary carbohydrates with unsaturated fatty acids in persons with the metabolic syndrome.

Aging. There is an increasing prevalence of the metabolic syndrome with advancing age.[41] This is true both in men and women. The association between age and the metabolic syndrome probably is due to multiple factors: higher obesity, reduced physical activity, decline in skeletal muscle mass, and decline in beta-cell function. The rise of blood pressure with aging likely is multifactorial in origin. Whether "cellular aging" enhances the metabolic risk factors is uncertain, but it may play a role.

Clinical consequences of the metabolic syndrome. The clinical consequences of the metabolic syndrome are several and common. The following diseases have been reported to be more common in patients with the metabolic syndrome:

- Coronary heart disease
- Stroke

- Type 2 diabetes
- Chronic renal failure
- Cholesterol gallstones
- Non-alcoholic fatty liver
- Cancer (?)

Clinical diagnosis. ATP III proposed a specific definition of the metabolic syndrome for use in clinical practice. Accordingly the metabolic syndrome is identified by the presence of three or more of the components listed in Table 4.

Prevalence of clinical metabolic syndrome. Recently Ford et al.[42] analyzed 8814 men and women over age 20 from the Third National Health and Nutrition Examination Survey (1988-1994) (NHANES III) to determine the prevalence of the metabolic syndrome as defined by ATP III. The overall prevalence of the metabolic syndrome in the United States was estimated to be 23.7%. After age 60, prevalence had increased to about 43.5% of the population, and the prevalence was similar for men and women for the whole population. However, in African Americans and Mexican Americans, the prevalence was higher in women than in men. According to this study, approximately 47 million US residents have the metabolic syndrome.

Approximately one-third of this number will have type 2 diabetes.

Laboratory reinforcement of diagnosis of metabolic syndrome: role of emerging risk factors. If more than three of the clinical abnormalities listed in Table 4 are detected, the diagnosis of the metabolic syndrome will be reinforced. Moreover, many patients with the metabolic syndrome have abnormalities in other emerging risk factors that are not detected in routine clinical evaluation. If testing is done for these risk factors and if abnormalities are detected, their presence will reinforce

Table 4–Clinical Identification of the Metabolic Syndrome

Risk Factor	Defining Level

Abdominal Obesity*
   Men
   Women
	Waist Circumference†
	 >102 cm (>40 in)
	 >88 cm (>35 in)

Triglycerides	≥150 mg/dL

HDL cholesterol
   Men
   Women
	
	 <40 mg/dL
	 <50 mg/dL

Blood pressure	≥130/≥85 mmHg
Fasting glucose	≥110 mg/dL

* Overweight and obesity are associated with insulin resistance and the metabolic syndrome. However, the presence of abdominal obesity is more highly correlated with the metabolic risk factors than is an elevated BMI. Therefore, the simple measure of waist circumference is recommended to identify the body weight component of the metabolic syndrome.

† Some male patients can develop multiple metabolic risk factors when the waist circumference is only marginally increased, e.g., 94-102 cm (37-39 in). Such patients may have a strong genetic contribution to insulin resistance. They should benefit from changes in life habits, similarly to men with categorical increases in waist circumference.

the diagnosis. However, their absence does not rule out the diagnosis if the essential criteria are present. These tests must be considered as optional for diagnosis reinforcement; several of these abnormalities however may be considered as direct targets for risk-reducing therapy. Other emerging risk factors that are manifestations of the basic metabolic-risk factors are the following:

- Atherogenic dyslipidemia
  - Small LDL particles
  - Small HDL particles
  - Elevated total apolipoprotein B

- Insulin resistance
  - Hyperinsulinemia
  - Impaired glucose tolerance
  - Fatty liver

- Prothrombotic state
  - Elevated PAI-1 levels
  - Elevated fibrinogen levels

- Proinflammatory state
  - Elevated hs-CRP
  - Elevated cytokines
  - Elevated Lp(a)
  - High homocysteine

Potential targets of therapy. The metabolic syndrome is a multiplex-risk factor, i.e., it consists of multiple metabolic risk factors. A fundamental question about the treatment of the metabolic syndrome is whether it is possible to employ a single therapeutic modality to modify the root causes of the syndrome, or whether it will be necessary to treat each of the individual risk factors separately. At present, the root causes of the metabolic syndrome are not fully understood. However, underlying risk factors for the metabolic syndrome are known, and these can be considered to be the primary targets of treatment. They include the following:

- Genetic susceptibility
- Overweight/obesity (especially abdominal obesity)
- Physical inactivity

Secondary targets of therapy in patients with the metabolic syndrome are the emerging risk factors. They are the following:

- Atherogenic dyslipidemia
- Elevated blood pressure
- Elevated plasma glucose
- Prothrombotic state
- Proinflammatory state

The approach to each of these risk factors will be described in more detail in subsequent sections on therapy.

Priority of Therapy: LDL First, Metabolic Syndrome Second

LDL CHOLESTEROL: PRIMARY TARGET OF THERAPY

In ATP III, elevations of serum LDL cholesterol constitute the primary target of therapy. For this reason, initiation of LDL-lowering therapy should precede other risk-reducing therapies directed to lipid-related targets. Of course, efforts to treat other major-risk factors—cigarette smoking, hypertension, and diabetes—must proceed in parallel with management of elevated LDL cholesterol. Nevertheless, initiation of management of other lipid-risk factors, underlying risk factors, and emerging risk factors should be delayed while primary attention is given to attaining the goals for LDL cholesterol. This recommendation is based on the principle of putting first things first.

ATP III proposes that three months of LDL-lowering therapy should be employed before turning to management of other metabolic risk factors. For primary prevention, this three-month period typically is devoted to dietary change designed to lower LDL levels. Thereafter, if necessary, LDL-lowering drugs can be added. In high-risk patients, however, it may be necessary to start drug therapy simultaneously with dietary change.

TREATMENT OF METABOLIC SYNDROME: BENEFIT BEYOND LDL LOWERING

After three months of LDL-lowering therapy, attention shifts to the metabolic syndrome—the secondary target of treatment. In some cases, treatment of metabolic syndrome will begin simultaneously with LDL-lowering drugs. Management of the metabolic syndrome has a two-fold aim. First attention is given to the underlying risk factors—overweight/obesity and physical inactivity. Second, if necessary, drug therapy can be considered to treat risk factors associated with the metabolic syndrome—hypertension, prothrombotic state, and atherogenic dyslipidemia. ATP III places more emphasis on the metabolic syndrome because of its growing prevalence in the US population and because its presence threatens to undo some of the benefit obtained from LDL-lowering therapy.

Therapeutic Modalities: Therapeutic Lifestyle Changes and Drug Therapy

ATP III offers two approaches to risk reduction. Therapeutic lifestyle changes (TLC) consist of a series on non-drug approaches to risk reduction. They are designed to lower LDL-cholesterol levels and to favorably modify the metabolic syndrome. When lifestyle therapies are insufficient to achieve recommended treatment goals, drug therapy can be introduced. The essential features of these two approaches will be outlined.

THERAPEUTIC LIFESTYLE CHANGES

The major components of lifestyle therapies in ATP III are:

LDL-Lowering Modalities

- Reduced intakes of saturated fats and cholesterol

- Therapeutic options for enhanced LDL
  lowering (plant stanol/sterols) and/or
  viscous fiber

The specific macronutrient recommendations of
the TLC diet are the following:

Nutrient	Recommended Intake
Saturated fat*	Less than 7% of total calories
Polyunsaturated fat	Up to 10% of total calories
Monounsaturated fat	Up to 20% of total calories
Total fat	25-35% of total calories
Carbohydrate† Fiber	50 to 60% of total calories 20-30 grams per day
Protein	Approximately 15% of total calories
Cholesterol	Less than 200 mg/day
Total calories (energy)‡	Balance energy intake and expenditure to maintain desirable body weight/prevent weight gain

*Trans fatty acids are another LDL-raising fat that should be kept
 at a low intake.
†Carbohydrate should be derived predominantly from foods rich
 in complex carbohydrates including grains, especially whole
 grains, fruits, and vegetables.
‡Daily energy expenditure should include at least moderate physical activity (contributing approximately 200 Kcal per day).

Metabolic Syndrome Therapies

- Weight reduction (also lowers LDL cholesterol)
- Increased physical activity

Anti-Atherogenic Diet: Other Dietary Changes to Reduce Baseline Risk

The overall composition of the TLC Diet is consistent with the recommendations of the Dietary Guidelines for Americans 2000, which lists its recommendations as follows:

Aim for Fitness

- Aim for a healthy weight
- Be physically active each day

Build a Healthy Dietary Base

- Let the food pyramid guide your food choices
- Choose a variety of grains daily, especially whole grains
- Choose a variety of fruits and vegetables daily
- Keep foods safe to eat

Choose Sensibly

- Choose a diet that is low in saturated fat and cholesterol and moderate in total fat
- Choose beverages and foods to moderate your intake of sugars
- Choose and prepare foods with less salt
- If you drink alcoholic beverages, do so in moderation

LDL-Lowering Approaches

Many reports reveal that there is a dose response relationship between intakes of saturated fatty acids and LDL-cholesterol levels. Diets high in saturated fatty acids raise serum LDL cholesterol, whereas reduction in intakes of saturated fatty acids lowers LDL cholesterol. Moreover, high intakes of saturated fatty acids are accompanied by high population rates of CHD. Conversely, clinical trials show that reduction in intake of saturated fatty acids will reduce risk for CHD. For these reasons, ATP III recommends that the TLC diet contain less than 7% of total calories as saturated fatty acids.

In addition, a review of the literature revealed that higher intakes of dietary cholesterol raise serum LDL-cholesterol levels in humans. Through this mechanism, higher intakes of dietary cholesterol likewise should raise the risk for CHD. By the same token, reducing cholesterol intakes from high to low decreases LDL cholesterol in most persons. Consequently, ATP III recommends that less than 200 mg per day of cholesterol should be consumed to maximize the amount of LDL-cholesterol-lowering that can be achieved through reduction in dietary cholesterol.

It must be noted that weight reduction, which is recommended primarily for treatment of the metabolic syndrome, will also lower LDL levels in some people. Weight reduction, of even a few pounds, may reduce LDL levels regardless of the nutrient composition of the weight loss diet; but weight reduction achieved through an energy-controlled diet low in saturated fatty acids and cholesterol often will enhance and sustain LDL-cholesterol-lowering.

Recent studies have shown that relatively low intakes of supplemental plant stanols or sterols will give additional LDL lowering. Daily intakes of 2 grams per day of plant stanol/sterols will reduce LDL cholesterol by 6-15%. Thus, plant stanol/sterols (2 g/day) are a therapeutic option to enhance LDL-cholesterol-lowering.

Moreover, adding 5-10 grams of viscous fiber per day to the diet will reduce LDL-cholesterol levels by approximately 5%. Thus daily use of dietary sources of viscous fiber is a therapeutic option to enhance LDL-cholesterol-lowering.

Finally, high intakes of soy protein can cause small reductions in LDL cholesterol, especially when they replace animal food products; thus food sources containing soy protein are acceptable as replacements for animal food products, particularly when the latter contain animal fats.

Lifestyle Therapies for the Metabolic Syndrome

After maximum reduction of LDL cholesterol with dietary therapy, emphasis shifts to management of the metabolic syndrome and associated lipid-risk factors. The majority of persons with these latter abnormalities are overweight or obese and sedentary. First-line therapies for all lipid and non-lipid-risk factors associated with the metabolic syndrome are weight reduction and increased physical activity, which will effectively reduce all of the associated risk factors. Therefore, after appropriate control of LDL cholesterol, TLC should stress weight reduction and physical activity if the metabolic syndrome is present.

In ATP III overweight and obesity are recognized as major, underlying risk factors for CHD and identified as direct targets of intervention. Weight reduction will enhance LDL lowering and reduce all of the risk factors of the metabolic syndrome. Assistance in the management of overweight and obese persons is provided by the Clinical Guidelines on the Identification, Evaluation, and Treatment of Overweight and Obesity in Adults from the NHLBI Obesity Education Initiative (1998).[24]

Physical inactivity is likewise a major, underlying risk factor for CHD. It augments the lipid and non-lipid-risk factors of the metabolic syndrome. It further may enhance risk by impairing cardiovascular fitness and coronary blood flow. Regular physical activity reduces VLDL levels, raises HDL cholesterol, and in some persons, lowers LDL levels. It also can lower blood pressure, reduce insulin resistance, and favorably influence cardiovascular function. ATP III thus recommends that regular physical activity become a routine component in management of high serum cholesterol. The evidence base for this recommendation is contained in the U.S. Surgeon General's Report on Physical Activity.[43]

Anti-Atherogenic Diet: Other Dietary Changes to Reduce Baseline Risk for CHD

Population baseline risk appears to be affected by lifestyle factors beyond LDL-raising nutrients, overweight/obesity, and physical inactivity. ATP III examined various dietary factors that may influence atherogenesis independently of these factors. The following summarizes the evidence and recommendations for several of these factors.

Trans Fatty Acids

Several reports indicate that *trans* fatty acids raise serum LDL-cholesterol levels and thus should increase risk for CHD. Some prospective studies support this conclusion. However, in ATP III, *trans* fatty acids are not classified as saturated fatty acids and are not included in the recommendation for saturated fatty acid intakes of <7% of calories in the TLC diet. Intakes of *trans* fatty acids nonetheless should be kept low by use of margarines low in these fatty acids.

Monounsaturated Fatty Acids

Metabolic studies show that these fatty acids lower LDL cholesterol when they replace saturated fatty acids in the diet. They do not lower HDL cholesterol nor do they raise triglycerides. Epidemiological studies further reveal that diets that contain substantial quantities of monounsaturated fatty acids from vegetable sources are associated with relatively low risks for CHD. ATP III therefore recommends that monounsaturated fatty acids be one form of unsaturated fatty acid to replace saturated fatty acids in the diet. They should be derived largely from plant sources. Intakes can range up to 20% of total calories.

Polyunsaturated Fatty Acids

The major polyunsaturated fatty acid is linoleic acid, which is derived largely from plant sources. Linoleic acid also reduces LDL cholesterol when it is substituted for saturated fatty acids in the diet. They also can produce small reductions in HDL cholesterol, compared with monounsaturated fatty acids. Several controlled clinical trials indicate that replacement of saturated acids with polyunsaturated fatty acids will reduce risk for CHD. Thus polyunsaturated fatty acids are one form of unsaturated fatty acids that can be used to replace saturated fatty acids in the diet. Intakes can range up to 10% of total energy.

Total Fat

Although "low fat" diets are widely recommended, higher intakes of total dietary fat, when composed mainly of unsaturated fatty acids, do not raise LDL cholesterol, compared to higher intakes of carbohydrate. For this reason, total fat does not require restriction for the purpose of lowering LDL cholesterol, provided that saturated fatty acids are reduced to the target goal. Furthermore, for persons with lipid disorders or the metabolic syndrome, extremes of fat intake—either high or low—should be avoided. When the metabolic syndrome is present, a total fat intake of 30-35% may reduce lipid and non-lipid-risk factors. The ATP III panel further supported the conclusions of the Dietary Guidelines for Americans 2000 that current evidence does not support the concept that the percentage of total fat in the diet, independent of caloric intake, is related to body weight or risk for cancer in the general population.

Carbohydrates

Replacement of saturated fatty acids with carbohydrates produces a fall in LDL-cholesterol levels. However, when intakes of carbohydrates are high (>60% of calories), HDL-cholesterol levels usually fall and triglycerides rise. For these reasons, carbohydrate intakes should be limited to 60% of total calories in persons with the metabolic syndrome. Moreover, lower intakes (e.g., 50% of calories) should be considered for persons with elevated triglycerides or low HDL cholesterol.

N-3 (omega-3) Polyunsaturated Fatty Acids

Several prospective studies and clinical trials suggest that higher intakes of n-3 fatty acids will reduce risk for coronary events or coronary mortality. The mechanisms whereby n-3 fatty acids might reduce coronary events are unknown and may be multiple. On the basis of this information, ATP III concluded that higher dietary intakes of n-3 fatty acids in the form of fatty fish or vegetable oils are an option for reducing risk for CHD. However, the recommendation for increased intakes of n-3 fatty acids was made optional because the strength of the evidence is only moderate.

Folic Acid and Vitamins B6 and B12

These vitamins have been claimed by some investigators to be anti-atherogenic. For example, they have been shown to reduce elevated levels of homocysteine, an emerging risk factor, in some persons. However, there are no published randomized controlled clinical trials to show whether lowering homocysteine levels through dietary intake or supplements of folate or other B vitamins will reduce risk for CHD. Regardless, ATP III endorsed the current RDA for dietary folate, namely, 400 micrograms per day.

DRUG THERAPY

Although therapeutic lifestyle changes are first-line therapy for cholesterol disorders, drug therapy may be required to achieve treatment goals for LDL cholesterol. Except for people with CHD and CHD risk equivalents, lifestyle therapies to reduce LDL cholesterol should always precede drug treatment. A 3-month trial of dietary therapy to lower LDL cholesterol is usually indicated before turning to drugs. The crite-

ria for consideration of drug therapy are outlined in the ATP III treatment algorithms. A few
comments about the rationale for selection of
specific drugs is warranted.

HMG CoA Reductase Inhibitors (Statins)

Overview. The statins. They are powerful cholesterol-lowering drugs that have proven to be
remarkably safe in clinical practice. Clinical trials have demonstrated that statins significantly
reduce the risk for CHD. The results of these
trials underlie the widespread use of these drugs
in high-risk patients.

Available statins. At present five statins are
available for use in clinical practice. These are:

- Lovastatin

- Pravastatin

- Simvastatin

- Fluvastatin

- Atorvastatin

One statin, cerivastatin, was recently withdrawn
by the manufacturer because of an increased frequency of side effects. Another statin, resuva-
statin, is in the later stages of development but
has not yet been approved by the Food and
Drug Administration for use in clinical practice.
Other statins reportedly are in development.

Mechanism of action. The primary action of statins is to reduce the synthesis of cholesterol by inhibiting HMG CoA reductase.[44,45] Most of this action occurs in the liver. By inhibiting the synthesis of cholesterol, statins reduce the cholesterol content of liver cells. The major consequence of this reduction is an increase in the expression of LDL receptors. These receptors are expressed on the surface of liver cells and facilitate uptake of plasma LDL and other apo B-containing lipoproteins by the liver. Among the latter are remnant lipoproteins. At high doses the statins appear to reduce the secretion of lipoproteins by the liver. Recent studies suggest that the increased expression of LDL receptors in the liver trap apo B-containing lipoproteins either within liver cells or within the space of Disse. These effects lead to a reduction in amounts of apo B-containing lipoproteins exiting the liver.

The dose-response relationship between statin dose and LDL lowering is hyperbolic. A simple relation has been noted, namely, for every doubling of the dose of statins, LDL cholesterol concentrations are reduced by 6%. According to this relationship, a tripling of the dose of statins lowers LDL-cholesterol levels by about 12%. This relation holds for all the statins. However, for a given weight of statin, LDL-lowering capacity differs. This fact requires that different doses of statins are needed to produce the same LDL lowering. The following lists what can be considered to be the "standard" dose for each of the statins, i.e., doses that produces approximately equivalent LDL lowering. This "standard" dose yields an approximate 30-35% reduction in LDL-cholesterol concentrations.

- Lovastatin   40 mg
- Pravastatin   40 mg
- Simvastatin   20 mg
- Fluvastatin   80 mg
- Atorvastatin   10 mg
- Rosuvastatin*   5 mg

Several reports suggest that statins have actions that appear to be unrelated to LDL lowering per se. These other actions have been called the *pleiotropic effects* of statin therapy. Notable among these are an anti-inflammatory response, antithrombotic tendency, reduced cellular proliferation, and improved vascular reactivity. Whether these responses are secondary to LDL lowering, reduction of other lipoproteins, inhibition of HMG CoA reductase, or other

*Rosuvastatin is currently under review by the FDA.

action has not been determined. Some investigators emphasize the importance of these pleiotropic effects and postulate that they contribute to the anti-atherogenic actions of these drugs. However, the major benefit of statin therapy appears to result from plasma lipid lowering.

Side effects. A variety of side effects have been attributed to statins. Early concerns that statins might cause cataracts have been ruled out by careful studies. Several other side effects have been reported in patients receiving statins:

- Gastrointestinal distress
- Skin reactions/allergic reactions
- Insomnia
- Elevated hepatic transaminases
- Myopathy

A few patients experience gastrointestinal distress, e.g., diarrhea. Rarely do gastrointestinal side effects require discontinuation of therapy. Skin and/or allergic reactions likewise can occur and require discontinuation; sometimes but not always changing to a different statin can avoid these reactions. There has been a dispute whether statins can induce insomnia. Data from clinical trials do not confirm a higher frequency of insomnia in patients treated with statins compared to controls; however, a few individuals report a strong relationship between statin ingestion and symptoms of insomnia. For patients who complain of insomnia, taking the statin in the morning instead of in the evening may reduce this symptom.

Without doubt, some patients who receive statins will experience an elevation of serum transaminases. This response has been considered by some investigators to reflect hepatotoxicity. However, there are no valid reports of patients developing severe hepatotoxicity and liver failure in which statins are clearly implicated. Furthermore, statins have not been implicated in the development of cirrhosis of the liver. Thus, modest-to-moderate rises in hepatic transaminases may be a physiological response to statins rather than a pathological response, and intensive routine monitoring of transaminases in patients on statin therapy appears to be unnecessary.

The major side effect of statins is myopathy. This condition occurs in various degrees of severity, which can be classified as follows:

- Mild myopathy
  - Myalgia without elevated creatine kinase (CK)

- Mild elevations of CK (<3 times normal)
  with or without myalgia
- Moderate myopathy
  - Myalgia plus moderate elevations of CK
    (3-10 times normal)
- Severe myopathy
  - Muscle pain and weakness plus severe
    elevations of CK (>10 times normal)

Mild myopathies in patients on statin therapy are relatively common. However, whether there is a cause-and-effect relationship is controversial. In controlled clinical trials, myalgias occur with similar frequency in placebo and drug-treatment groups. Nonetheless, in clinical practice, a few patients complain of myalgias that are temporally related to statin use. The approach to such patients can vary, but consideration can be given to reducing the dose to the minimally tolerable dose; thereafter, the dose can be gradually increased as tolerated. Switching to another statin may reduce the myalgia. Anecdotal reports suggest that various supplements (co-enzyme Q-10 and L-carnitine) reduce myalgias accompanying statin therapy, but the benefit may be attributed to placebo effect in some patients.

Moderate myopathy can be treated similarly to milder forms. However, if serum CK levels remain substantially elevated, reducing the dose or stopping the drug may be necessary. Some individuals have a high baseline of CK and can tolerate statins without harm; therefore, a baseline measurement of CK is useful to identify those who habitually run high levels. It must also be remembered that mild forms of trauma can raise CK levels, and when elevations are found in patients taking statins, careful questioning for recent traumatic episodes should be pursued.

Severe myopathy occurs infrequently but can have serious consequences. This condition is accompanied by muscle pain and weakness and CK levels >10-fold elevated. The greatest concern is myoglobinuria resulting in acute renal failure. Occasionally, patients with severe myopathy will die from acute renal failure. Recently cerivastatin was removed from the market because of an excessive risk for severe myopathy. With other statins, about one person in 1000 treated with statins will develop severe myopathy. Most persons who develop severe myopathy have risk factors for this condition. Physicians should be aware of the risk factors for severe myopathy and when possible statins should either be avoided or the dose should be kept low.

In 2001, the Bayer company voluntarily withdrew cerivastatin from the market because of an unacceptably high frequency of myopathy and the rarer severe myopathy (rhabdomyolysis) associated with cerivastatin therapy. The risk was particularly high when cerivastatin was used concomitantly with gemfibrozil. The FDA recently reviewed U.S. reports to the FDA associated with all statin drugs and published their findings in a letter to the *New England Journal of Medicine*.[46] Fatal severe myopathy was found to be a rare event occurring with statin therapy; less than 1 death per million prescriptions was reported. Seemingly, the rate of fatal severe myopathy with cerivastatin therapy was 16-80 times higher than reported for other statins. Although rates of reporting may have underestimated the true incidence of severe myopathy, it was clear that cerivastatin stood out as being particularly dangerous compared to the other statins. To a large extent, the findings reported in this letter were reassuring regarding the low risk of severe myopathy accompanying the other statins. Nonetheless, severe (and fatal) myopathy has been reported for all of the statins; this emphasizes the need to use and monitor statins appropriately for the clinical condition of the patient.

The following groups are at higher risk for severe myopathy: older people, especially those with multi-system disease (e.g., chronic renal insufficiency) or those who are frail with small body frame; patients taking multiple medications, particularly fibrates, cyclosporine, azole antifungals, intraconazole and ketoconazole, macrolide antibiotics, erythromycin and clarithromycin, HIV protease inhibitors, the antidepressant Netazodone, and verapamil; surgery patients during perioperative periods; and persons who consume large quantities of grapefruit juice (e.g., >1 quart per day) or who abuse alcohol. It usually is advisable to withhold statin therapy when patients are admitted to the hospital for acute illnesses or for major surgery.

Clinical trials of statin therapy. Several landmark clinical trials have been carried out with statin therapy. On the whole, these trials show that statin therapy reduces risk for acute coronary syndromes, coronary procedures, and other coronary outcomes in both primary and secondary prevention. Statins also reduce stroke incidence in patients with established CHD. Thus, statins can be considered first-line drugs for management of elevated LDL cholesterol. The benefit of statin therapy has been confirmed in six major clinical trials. The results of each trial can be reviewed briefly.

Scandinavian Simvastatin Survival Study (4S)[11] was a secondary prevention trial; the effect of therapy with simvastatin on total mortality was assessed in 4,444 patients with CHD and baseline total cholesterol 212-309 mg/dL. The trial was a multicenter, randomized, double-blind, placebo-controlled study. Patients were treated with standard care, including diet, and either simvastatin 20-40 mg/day (n=2,221) or placebo (n=2,223) for a median duration of 5.4 years. Over the course of the study, treatment with simvastatin led to mean reductions in total-C, LDL-C and TG of 25%, 35%, and 10% respectively, and a mean increase in HDL-C of 8%. Simvastatin significantly reduced the risk of mortality by 30%, (p=0.0003, 182 deaths in the simvastatin group vs. 256 deaths in the placebo group). The risk of CHD mortality was significantly reduced by 42%, (p=0.00001, 111 vs. 189 deaths). The risk of major coronary events was significantly reduced by 34%, (p<0.00001, 431 vs. 622 patients with one or more events). The risk of a hospital-verified nonfatal MI was reduced by 37%. Simvastatin also significantly reduced the risk of undergoing myocardial revascularization procedures (PTCA, CABG) by 37%, (p<0.00001, 252 vs. 383 patients). And simvastatin significantly reduced the risk of fatal and nonfatal cerebrovascular events (combined stroke and transient ischemic attacks) by 28% (p=0.033, 75 vs. 102 patients).

The 4S study was an extremely important clinical trial that made several important contributions to the field. It showed that effective LDL-lowering therapy markedly reduces risk for both major coronary events and even stroke. Of great importance, 4S demonstrated that LDL-lowering therapy decreases total mortality. This finding proves conclusively that side effects of cholesterol lowering do not outweigh the benefits. Statin therapy in patients with established CHD was shown to be highly cost-effective compared to other forms of medical therapy. 4S was the first of several landmark statin trials to follow.

The Cholesterol and Recurrent Events Study (CARE)[12] was a secondary prevention trial using pravastatin to treat coronary patients with relatively normal cholesterol levels. The effect of pravastatin, 40 mg daily, on coronary heart disease death and nonfatal MI was assessed in 4,159 patients who had experienced a myocardial infarction in the preceding 3-20 months and who had normal (below the 75th percentile of the general population) plasma total cholesterol levels. Pravastatin therapy lowered LDL cholesterol to an average level of 98 mg/dL. With this response, major coronary events decreased by 24%. Treatment with pravastatin significantly reduced the rate of first recurrent coronary events (either CHD death or nonfatal MI), the risk of undergoing revascularization procedures (PTCA, CABG), and the risk of stroke or transient ischemic attack.

The CARE trial confirmed the benefit of LDL-lowering therapy in patients with established CHD. It showed that CHD risk is significantly lowered even when patients with established CHD do not have elevated LDL cholesterol at baseline. CARE investigators have carried out a large number of subgroup analyses of this study. One controversial outcome of the CARE study was its inability to document benefit of LDL-lowering therapy when (a) baseline LDL cholesterol was <125 mg/dL, or (b) LDL cholesterol was reduced to <125 mg/dL.[47] On the other hand, it demonstrated CHD risk reduction in patients with type 2 diabetes.[48]

The Long-Term Intervention with Pravastatin in Ischemic Disease (LIPID)[13] assessed the effect of pravastatin, 40 mg daily, in 9,014 patients who had experienced either an MI (5,754 patients) or had been hospitalized for unstable angina pectoris (3,260 patients) in the preceding 3-36 months.

Patients in this multi-center, double-blind, placebo-controlled study participated for an average of 5.6 years (median of 5.9 years) and at randomization had total cholesterol between 114 and 563 mg/dL (mean 219 mg/dL), LDL-C between 46 and 274 mg/dL (mean 150 mg/dL), triglycerides between 35 and 2,710 mg/dL (mean 160 mg/dL), and HDL-C between 1 and 103 mg/dL (mean 37 mg/dL). At baseline, 82% of patients were receiving aspirin and 76% were receiving antihypertensive medication. Treatment with pravastatin significantly reduced the risk of total mortality (by reducing CHD death) and CHD events (CHD mortality or nonfatal MI). The reduction in CHD mortality was consistent regardless of age.

The LIPID study extended the two preceding secondary prevention trials with statin therapy. LIPID confirmed reduction in major coronary events and stroke, and it also confirmed a reduction in CHD mortality. Analysis of the trial also found no heterogeneity in beneficial responses among different subgroups categorized according to age, sex, hypertension, or diabetes. Like CARE, LIPID detected no benefit of statin therapy in patients with low LDL cholesterol levels, i.e., <125 mg/dL.

Recently the investigators of CARE and LIPID have pooled their data on pravastatin therapy to enhance the power of post hoc analysis. When the data from CARE and LIPID were combined, the pooled data still failed to reveal a significant reduction in risk for major coronary events in patients with low baseline LDL cholesterol (i.e., <125 mg/dL).[49] However, in CHD patients with diabetes, a significant reduction in major coronary events was observed in those with low baseline LDL cholesterol. This finding suggests that statin therapy may be more efficacious in CHD patients who have other lipid-risk factors, such as low HDL cholesterol and high triglycerides.

The West of Scotland Coronary Prevention Study (WOSCOPS), a primary prevention trial, was conducted on hypercholesterolemic patients with a mean (±SD) plasma cholesterol level of 272 ±23 mg/dL.[14] On the basis of risk factor status, most enrollees fell into the moderately high-risk category. Patients received pravastatin therapy (40 mg daily) or placebo. The average follow-up period was 4.9 years. Pravastatin lowered plasma cholesterol levels by 20% and LDL cholesterol levels by 26%; there was no change in the placebo group. Reduced cholesterol levels in the pravastatin group were accompanied by a 31% decrease in major coronary events. There were similar reductions in the risk of definite nonfatal myocardial infarctions, death from coronary heart disease, and death from all cardiovascular causes. There was no excess of death from noncardiovascular causes. An overall 22% reduction in the risk of death from any cause was observed in the pravastatin group.

WOSCOPS was the first large primary prevention trial with statin therapy. It extended the benefit of statins to patients without established CHD. Patients in WOSCOPS generally were hypercholesterolemic and had a moderately high risk (average 10 year risk for major coronary events about 15%).

The Air Force/Texas Coronary Atherosclerosis Prevention Study (AFCAPS/ TexCAPS) also was a primary prevention study; a randomized, double-blind, placebo-controlled trial, it included 6,605 men and women without established CHD who had average total cholesterol and LDL cholesterol and below average HDL cholesterol. Treatment with lovastatin 20-40 mg/day resulted in a 25% reduction in LDL cholesterol and a 6% increase in HDL cholesterol, and produced a 37% reduction in risk of a first acute major coronary event, defined as fatal or nonfatal myocardial infarction, unstable angina, or sudden cardiac death.[15]

AFCAPS/TexCAPS extended the benefits of statins to primary prevention in moderate risk patients. Absolute risk for major coronary events was about 7% per 10 years. The reduction in relative risk with statin therapy nonetheless was impressive; however, for those individuals at only moderate risk, the cost-effectiveness of statin therapy is open to some question. Thus AFCAPS/TexCAPS highlights the issue of cost-effectiveness and required this issue to be considered in detail by the ATP III panel.

Heart Protection Study (HPS). This study was carried out in the United Kingdom.[16] This study recruited about 20,000 high-risk patients who had a history of myocardial infarction or other CHD, occlusive disease of non-coronary arteries, or diabetes mellitus or hypertension. Subjects were men and women ranging in age from 40-80 years. All patients had a total cholesterol >3.5 mmol/L (>135 mg/dL). The trial tested statin and mixed antioxidant vitamins and their use was not considered clearly indicated or contraindicated by the patients' own physicians. Four arms of the study included simvastatin (40 mg daily) vs. placebo and vitamins (600 mg vitamin E, 250 mg vitamin C, and 20 mg beta-carotene vs. placebo.) The study's duration was 5 years. At the end, no benefit was observed with vitamin therapy for major cardiovascular events. In contrast, simvastatin therapy produced an across-the-board risk reduction for major coronary events, coronary procedures, stroke, and total mortality. All told, major cardiovascular events were reduced by about one quarter with simvastatin therapy. It was postulated by the researchers that an even greater benefit would have been achieved had not a significant portion of patients in the placebo groups been started on statin therapy by their personal physicians.

HPS results produced evidence of benefits of LDL-lowering therapy by statins in various subgroups who were high-risk at recruitment: patients with and without established CHD, patients with and without diabetes, older as well as younger patients, patients with non-coronary forms of atherosclerotic disease, and patients with borderline-high, near-optimal, and optimal levels of LDL cholesterol. This study thus appears to have important implications for cholesterol management in high-risk patients, although further analysis will be required for recommendations on adjustment of therapies in various patient subgroups.

Clinical usage. ATP III identified statins as first-line therapies for LDL lowering. Statins are particularly useful in high-risk patients. However, they are being employed increasingly in persons who are at intermediate risk, particularly in older persons. Statins are particularly valuable in patients with severe hypercholesterolemia. As the costs of statins decline, their usage in clinical practice undoubtedly will rise.

Bile Acid Sequestrants

Overview. Bile acid sequestrants have been used for many years as cholesterol-lowering therapy. The drugs bind bile acids, a cholesterol product, in the intestine. Although bile acid sequestrants have been largely superceded by statins, they nonetheless can be used as primary therapy in some patients and can be combined with statins to obtain enhanced LDL lowering in other patients.

Available drugs. There are three bile acid sequestrants available for cholesterol-lowering therapy:

- Cholestyramine
- Colestipol
- Colesevelam

Cholestyramine was the first bile acid sequestrant used in clinical practice. It is a powder and usual doses range from 8 to 16 g/day. Lower doses are better tolerated, but somewhat greater LDL reductions are obtained at higher doses. Colestipol is a similar drug for which doses range from 10 to 20 g/day. Recently a new bile acid sequestrant, colesevelam, was introduced. This drug binds bile acids much more avidly than older sequestrants; the usual dose is 3.6 g/day.

Mechanism of action. The sequestrants bind bile acids in the intestine and interrupt their enterohepatic circulation; as a result, the liver converts more cholesterol into bile acids. This drain on hepatic cholesterol enhances LDL-receptor activity and lowers LDL-cholesterol levels by 15-30%, depending on dose. At usual doses, LDL-cholesterol levels are reduced by 15-20%. These responses are additive to LDL reductions obtained by statins. For example, if a statin lowers LDL-cholesterol levels by 30%-35%, the addition of a bile acid sequestrant allows for a reduction of about 45%-50%.[51,52]

Side effects. Bile acid sequestrants remain exclusively in the gastrointestinal tract; likewise the major side effects are gastrointestinal. Some patients experience upper gastrointestinal distress, but the usual side effect is constipation. This side effect often abates over time. Moreover, it can be alleviated by use of bulk fiber, e.g., psyllium-based bulking agents.

Sequestrants can bind some drugs, and it is useful to separate timing of dosing with other drugs and sequestrants. Examples of drugs in which sequestrants can interfere with absorption are digitoxin, warfarin, thyroxine, thiazide diuretics, and beta-blockers.

Another side effect of bile acid sequestrants is a rise of serum triglycerides. The mechanism of this effect is not known. Bile acid sequestrants are particularly contraindicated in patients who have severe hypertriglyceridemia, and they generally are not recommended when triglycerides are moderately elevated. However, this should not be taken to mean that bile acid sequestrants are contraindicated in patients with type 2 diabetes; one study showed that these drugs are particularly effective in LDL lowering when patients have this form of diabetes.[53]

Clinical trials. The Lipid Research Clinics-Coronary Primary Prevention Trial (LRC-CPPT)[3] was a large clinical trial carried out in 3,806 middle-aged men with hypercholesterolemia who did not have established CHD. Study duration was 7.4 years. Compared to placebo, cholestyramine therapy lowered LDL-cholesterol levels by 12.6%. This reduction was accompanied by a 19% decrease in major coronary events (p <0.05). Other CHD endpoints also were reduced on cholestyramine therapy: new positive exercise tests by 25%, new angina pectoris by 20%, and coronary bypass surgery by 25%. Presumably because of the relatively small size of the groups under study and because of the relatively small reduction in LDL cholesterol, total mortality was not reduced. At the time of publication, skeptics were concerned that failure to find a reduction in total mortality indicated a lack of overall benefit of cholesterol-lowering therapy. However, the reduction in total mortality with the more powerful statin drugs has removed this doubt. It now is clear that the study was lacking in statistical power to test the total-mortality question.

Clinical usage. ATP III identified bile acid sequestrants as agents proven to reduce risk for CHD. Moreover, these drugs are additive in LDL lowering when used in combination with other drugs (e.g., statins). ATP III recommended that consideration be given to prescribing bile acid sequestrants for persons with moderate elevations of LDL cholesterol. They may be safer than statins for young adults or women who are considering pregnancy. They are particularly useful in persons with very high LDL-cholesterol concentrations when used in combination with statins.

One of the drawbacks of bile acid sequestrants has been the nuisance of their bulk. Many patients do not like to take 8-20 grams of powdered sequestrants daily. In addition, they often cause gastrointestinal distress including constipation. The problem of constipation can generally be overcome by combining sequestrants with bulking agents, but here again, more bulk is required. For this reason, there has been a growing interest in the use of agents that act in lower doses to block the absorption of bile acids. One class of agents that is currently under investigation includes bile-acid transport (BAT) inhibitors. Another approach has been to develop more efficacious bile acid sequestrants. The first drug in this class is colesevelam. When used alone, colesevelam in doses of about 3.6 gm/day reduces LDL cholesterol by 15-20%;[54-56] when combined with a statin, incremental reductions of 10-15% usually are obtained.

Cholesterol-Absorption Blockers

Another approach to reduction of LDL-cholesterol levels is to block the absorption of cholesterol. This approach has been recognized for many years, but until the benefits of LDL-lowering with statin therapy were documented, there was little interest in this approach. However, because of the success of statin therapy, we are living in a new age of interest in prevention of CHD through LDL lowering. Consequently, the possibility of obtaining incremental benefit by alternative mechanisms has received increased attention.

One modality for lowering of serum LDL-cholesterol concentrations by inhibiting the absorption of cholesterol is currently available. Plant stanols and plant sterols when given in a dose of about 2 gm/day will lower LDL-cholesterol levels in the range of 10-15%.[57,58] Plant stanols/sterols can be obtained in the form of margarines (trade names: Benecol and Take Control). Other vehicles for plant stanol/sterols are under development. These products can be used to enhance the LDL-lowering of dietary therapy,[1] or they can enhance efficacy of LDL lowering from statin therapy.[59] The potential of plant stanols/sterols to achieve greater reduction of CHD has been reviewed and put into perspective.[60,61] ATP III recommended consideration of plant stanols/sterols for patients who are already undergoing LDL-lowering therapy.[1] A more effective cholesterol-absorption blocker is ezetimibe; this agent selectively blocks the absorption of cholesterol when given in low doses. Clinical studies have shown that it will reduce LDL-cholesterol concentrations in the range of 15-20%;[62,63] to date, however, ezetimibe is still under development and has not yet been approved for use in clinical practice by the FDA.

Nicotinic Acid

Overview. Nicotinic acid also has long been used to treat hyperlipidemia. In low intakes, nicotinic acid is a vitamin; at high doses it acts as a LDL-lowering drug. High-dose nicotinic acid was first used to treat hypercholesterolemia; more recently, it was recognized that the major action of nicotinic acid is to lower serum triglyceride and to raise HDL cholesterol. Although nicotinic acid is a powerful lipid-altering drug, its use in clinical practice has been limited because of the side effects that often accompany high doses of the drug. This disparity has led to major efforts to develop dosage forms that will reduce the side effects.

Available drugs. Nicotinic acid is available in three forms:

- Crystalline nicotinic acid
- Sustained-release nicotinic acid
- Extended-release nicotinic acid (Niaspan®)

Crystalline nicotinic acid is inexpensive but has two disadvantages: it must be taken several times per day and in many people it is accompanied by unacceptable flushing of the skin. Sustained-release nicotinic acid reduces flushing, but is accompanied by increased hepatotoxicity. More recently, extended-release nicotinic acid (Niaspan®) has been introduced; this agent reduces flushing and hepatotoxicity compared to crystalline nicotinic acid.

Mechanism of action. To date the mechanism whereby nicotinic acid modifies lipoprotein metabolism is not well understood. Its major action appears to be to reduce the secretion of apo B-containing lipoproteins into the circulation. One action of nicotinic acid is inhibition of triglyceride lipolysis in adipose tissue; the resulting reduction in plasma non-esterified fatty acids (NEFA) could decrease the rate of synthesis of VLDL. Although this mechanism may pertain, it does not appear adequate to explain all of the actions of nicotinic acid. Seemingly nicotinic acid also acts in the liver to alter the assembly of triglyceride-rich lipoproteins (TGRLP). Another action of nicotinic acid is to cause a striking increase in HDL-cholesterol levels, and this apparently cannot be explained by reduced secretion of TGRLP. How nicotinic acid raises HDL is not known.

Side effects. Nicotinic acid has several side effects that make it unacceptable to about one-fourth of patients. These include flushing, itching, and rashes of the skin, gastrointestinal distress, hepatotoxicity, hyperuricemia, and hyperglycemia. Flushing is more frequent with crystalline nicotinic acid, whereas the sustained release form is more likely to cause hepatotoxicity. Extended release nicotinic acid (Niaspan®) causes less flushing than the crystalline form and causes less hepatotoxicity than sustained-release preparations.

Clinical trials. Two endpoint trials have been carried out with nicotinic acid: the Coronary Drug Project (CDP)[64] and the Stockholm Ischemic Heart Disease Study.[65] The CDP was a large secondary prevention study that compared several drugs including clofibrate and nicotinic acid for their efficacy in patients with established CHD. Treatment with nicotinic acid produced a significantly lower incidence of recurrence of major coronary events. The reduction in recurrence of CHD events was 25%. In long-term follow-up of CDP patients revealed that those who had received nicotinic acid during the trial had a reduction in total mortality.[66] In spite of this benefit, patients who received nicotinic acid also had a relatively high frequency of the side effects that are common with nicotinic acid therapy.

The Stockholm study[65] also was a secondary prevention trial. It combined clofibrate and nicotinic acid into a single drug regimen. The trial was relatively small (276 patients in the placebo group and 279 patients receiving drug therapy). Drug treatment reduced serum cholesterol and triglycerides by 13% and 17%, respectively. The group that received combined drug therapy had a 26% lower total mortality ($p < 0.05$), whereas CHD mortality was lowered by 36% ($p < 0.01$). Patients who had relatively high triglyceride levels at outset appeared to benefit most from therapy. Although the study was small, its result suggested that benefit of lipid-lowering therapy can be achieved in high-risk patients even when the therapy is not directed primarily towards LDL cholesterol.

Potential clinical usage. ATP III judges nicotinic acid to be a therapeutic option for high-risk persons with atherogenic dyslipidemia. It can be used as a single agent in people who are at or near their goals for LDL cholesterol. Nicotinic acid appears to be especially useful in combination therapy with other cholesterol-lowering drugs in high-risk persons in whom atherogenic dyslipidemia is combined with elevated

LDL-cholesterol levels. Nonetheless nicotinic acid should be used cautiously in patients with active liver disease, recent peptic ulcer, and hyperuricemia.

Since the introduction of Niaspan®, there has been a renewed interest in the use of nicotinic acid. This is because Niaspan® seems to be better tolerated than other forms of nicotinic acid. There apparently is less hepatotoxicity with Niaspan® than with sustained-release preparations. Niaspan® also causes less flushing than does crystalline nicotinic acid. It must be pointed out nonetheless that crystalline nicotinic acid is well-tolerated by many patients. 50-75% of patients treated with crystalline nicotinic acid seem to be able to tolerate it on a long-term basis.[67,68] A higher percentage, 75-85% apparently can maintain therapy with Niaspan®. In a word, crystalline nicotinic acid is less expensive but also less well tolerated than Niaspan®.[69,70] Several recent studies[69-71] have been reported in which Niaspan® was used alone or in combination with other lipid-lowering drugs.

Use of nicotinic acid in clinical practice requires commitment on the part of physicians as well as of patients. Drug therapy with nicotinic acid is best initiated at lower doses and titrated to higher doses. If crystalline nicotinic

acid is employed, doses can begin at 50 mg
three times per day and gradually increased to
500 mg three times per day or even up to
1000 mg three times per day. For Niaspan®,
the initial dose can be 500 mg/day with a final
dose of 1000-2000 mg/day. Niaspan® can be
given as a single dose at bedtime. Clinical
experience has shown that slow upward titra-
tion of nicotinic acid provides the best outcome
for acceptance and long-term adherence to
drug therapy.

An important question is whether nicotinic
acid can be used safely in patients with diabetes. Since type 2 diabetes is commonly
accompanied by atherogenic dyslipidemia,
nicotinic acid theoretically should be an ideal
agent to employ in patients with this form of
diabetes. In fact, the lipid and lipoprotein profile is greatly improved in patients with type 2
diabetes.[72] On the other hand, when nicotinic
acid is given in relatively high doses to these
patients, there is a worsening of glucose control.[72] Thus, high doses of nicotinic acid (e.g.,
3-4 gm/day) probably should not be used in
patients with diabetes. On the other hand, in
recent years, there has been a growing interest
in the use of lower doses of nicotinic acid for
this purpose. One report[73] indicated that crys-

talline nicotinic acid in doses of 1.5-3.0 gm/day can be used to effectively treat atherogenic dys-lipidemia in patients with diabetes without appreciably worsening glycemic control. Even more recently, Grundy et al.[74] reported that Niaspan® in doses of 1.0 to 1.5 gm/day improves atherogenic dyslipidemia in patients with type 2 diabetes without substantially worsening glucose control. When using nico-tinic acid as therapy in patients with type 2 diabetes, the best approach would appear to be to monitor $HbA1_c$ percentages. If the percent-age of $HbA1_c$ does not increase significantly during therapy, then nicotinic acid can be safe-ly continued.

There is a growing view among authorities that nicotinic acid therapy is best carried out in combination with statins. Studies have shown that this combination is highly efficacious for improving all lipoprotein fractions.[71] One new drug combination, Advicor®, which consists of Niaspan® + lovastatin has recently been approved by the Food and Drug Adminis-tration. This drug combination appears to be promising to achieve LDL-cholesterol targets plus improvement of atherogenic dyslipidemia. The goal of therapy is to achieve incremental risk reduction beyond what can be achieved by use of a statin alone. Although combined drug therapy has not been extensively tested in large clinical end-point trials, results obtained in angiographic studies are highly suggestive of incremental benefit from combinations of lipid-lowering drugs.[75,76]

Fibric Acid Derivatives (Fibrates)

Overview. Fibrates have been used for almost four decades for treatment of hyperlipidemia. A large body of data has been obtained on their actions, and several clinical trials provide evidence of CHD risk reduction. Interest in fibrates has grown in the past few years because of new information of their mechanisms of action.

Available drugs. Four fibrates are being used for lipid-lowering. They are the following:

- Gemfibrozil
- Fenofibrate
- Bezafibrate
- Clofibrate

Gemfibrozil is the major fibrate being used in the United States. However, there is a growing use of fenofibrate. Bezafibrate is available in several other countries, but not in the United States. Clofibrate is available, but rarely is used.

Mechanisms of action. Fibrates have been found to have a variety of actions. These include increased oxidation of fatty acids in the liver, decreased synthesis of apolipoprotein CIII, increased activity of lipoprotein lipase, increased production of apolipoprotein AI, decreased synthesis of bile acids, and increased secretion of cholesterol into bile. For many years these pleiotropic effects could not be explained. The critical link to mechanism of action was the discovery that fibrates are agonists for nuclear receptors called peroxisomal proliferation activation receptor (PPAR) alpha. These nuclear receptors initiate a series of gene activations that account for the multiple physiological responses that are typical of fibrate action.[77,78]

Side effects. The side effects of fibrates are gastrointestinal distress, skin reactions, myopathy, and cholesterol gallstones. Myopathy with fibrate therapy is most likely to occur in patients with end-stage renal disease and when they are used in combination with statins. Cholesterol gallstones occur in 2-5% of patients receiving fibrates. Early clinical trials suggested that fibrates may increase non-CHD mortality; more recent clinical trials however have not confirmed this trend.

Clinical trials. Several primary and secondary prevention trials have been carried out with different fibrates. Five major trials can be briefly reviewed.

The World Health Organization (WHO) trial[79] tested clofibrate versus placebo in 15,745 men, ages 30 to 59 in the United Kingdom and Eastern Europe. This was a primary prevention trial. Treatment with clofibrate reduced total cholesterol levels by 9% and ischemic heart disease events by 20%. Further nonfatal myocardial infarction was reduced by 25%. In spite of clinical benefit, clofibrate therapy was accompanied by an overall increase in death rates, apparently due to diseases of the biliary and gastrointestinal tract. It is known that fibrates increase the incidence of cholesterol gallstones, and some of the excess of deaths may have been explained by complications of gallstone disease. Thus, in spite of a reduction in CHD rates, the specter of adverse effects with clofibrate in particular and fibrates in general subsequently limited enthusiasm for fibrate use in clinical practice.

Subsequently, the Helsinki Heart Study,[80] another primary prevention trial, randomized 4,061 asymptomatic, middle-aged men (ages 40 to 55 years) to either gemfibrozil therapy or placebo. Gemfibrozil therapy in this 5-year trial reduced major coronary events by 34% compared to placebo (P <0.02). This trial was not powered to test efficacy for reduction in total mortality, and total deaths were neither increased nor decreased with gemfibrozil therapy. Although no increase in total morality was observed, the failure to reduce total mortality with gemfibrozil therapy again dampened enthusiasm for fibrate therapy for primary prevention of CHD.

Three secondary prevention trials also have been carried out with fibrates. In the first of these, the Coronary Drug Project,[64] clofibrate therapy failed to reduce rates of recurrent CHD compared to placebo. In a second trial, the Bezafibrate Infarction Prevention Study (BIP), treatment of patients with established CHD with bezafibrate likewise failed to significantly reduce major coronary events compared to placebo. In contrast, a positive result was obtained in the Veterans Affairs HDL Intervention Trial (VA-HIT),[82] which compared gemfibrozil therapy to placebo in 2,500 men with established CHD. Treatment with gemfibrozil produced significant reductions in all coronary endpoints as well as in stroke. Overall risk for CHD was reduced by about 18%. It has been pointed out that BIP and VA-HIT trials differed in patient recruitment. BIP recruited mainly patients with higher

LDL-cholesterol levels who nowadays would be candidates for statin therapy. VA-HIT recruited patients who mainly had low LDL cholesterol, atherogenic dyslipidemia, and the metabolic syndrome. Consequently it has been speculated that if fibrates are effective they will be most efficacious in patients who have these latter disorders, largely those with the metabolic syndrome.

Although the fibrate trials taken together have given a mixed result, a pooling of all the data in meta-analysis have revealed that fibrates do in fact lower risk for major coronary events (see ATP III full report, www.nhlbi.nih.gov). Risk reduction is in the range of 15-20%, or about half of what is obtained with statin therapy. This reduction in CHD events in short-term clinical trials is insufficient to be reflected in a significant reduction in total mortality. However, in fibrate trials after the WHO study, no indication has surfaced for significant fibrate toxicity that increases the risk for death. Thus, clinical trial data leave open the possibility that fibrates may be useful as adjuncts with statin therapy for patients with atherogenic dyslipidemia and/or the metabolic syndrome. Finally, it should be noted that several angiographic trials have demonstrated that fibrate therapy can favorably modify coronary atherosclerotic lesions as studied by coronary angiography.[83-85]

Clinical usage. ATP III recommends that fibrates be considered for persons with very high triglyceride concentrations to reduce risk for acute pancreatitis. They also are useful in patients with dysbetalipoproteinemia (elevated beta-VLDL). Finally, they are an option for combination therapy with statins in persons who have both elevated LDL cholesterol and athero-genic dyslipidemia.

Other Agents

ATP III notes that high doses of N-3 polyunsatu-rated fatty acids lower triglyceride levels and thus can be used in patients with hypertriglyceridemia. However, more clinical trials remain necessary before N-3 fatty acids can be recommended rou-tinely for primary or secondary prevention. In ATP II, estrogen replacement therapy was sug-gested for treatment of elevated LDL cholesterol in postmenopausal women. However, because of recent negative coronary outcome trials with such therapy, postmenopausal estrogens are not recom-mended specifically for treatment of hypercholes-terolemia or for prevention of CHD. In contrast, ATP III notes that statin therapy is effective for lowering risk for coronary events in women with established CHD.

Management of LDL Cholesterol in Different Risk Categories

HIGH-RISK PATIENTS: CHD AND CHD RISK EQUIVALENTS

ATP III goals for LDL cholesterol in high-risk patients. Recent clinical trials have demonstrated that LDL-lowering therapy reduces total mortality, coronary mortality, major coronary events, coronary artery procedures, and strokes in persons with established CHD. Since an LDL-cholesterol level of <100 mg/dL is optimal, ATP III specifies an LDL cholesterol <100 mg/dL as the goal of therapy in patients with established CHD. A goal of <100 mg/dL is supported by clinical trials with both clinical and angiographic endpoints and by prospective epidemiological studies. This same goal is recommended for patients with CHD risk equivalents.

The question can be raised as to what is meant by the ATP III goal for LDL cholesterol of "less than 100 mg/dL" in high-risk patients. How much below 100 mg/dL should the LDL be lowered? This question has not been fully resolved. Clinical trials are currently underway to determine whether a lowering of LDL levels to well below 100 mg/dL will produce further risk reduction, and if so, by how much. The answer to these questions should be forthcoming within a few years. However, the recent results of the Heart Protection Study[16] may shed some additional light on the questions. A preliminary interpretation of the results of this study is provided in the following.

Relation between LDL-cholesterol levels and CHD risk in high-risk patients. The precise relation between LDL-cholesterol levels and CHD risk has been a topic of on-going discussion. On the basis of previous clinical trial data, the author[86] reviewed three hypotheses regarding the relationship: (a) linear, (b) curvilinear (log-linear), and (c) threshold (Figure 7). According to the first hypothesis, progressive lowering of LDL cholesterol results in a progressive lowering of CHD risk in a linear manner; the second hypothesis suggests a progressive lowering but with decreasing decrements in absolute risk

Figure 7 - Three models for the relationship between LDL cholesterol levels and relative risk for coronary heart disease. According to the linear model (A), relative risk declines linearly to LDL-cholesterol levels of 100 mg/dL and below. Model (B) shows a curvilinear (log-linear) relationship. Relative risk falls progressively with lower LDL-cholesterol levels, but benefit declines with lower and lower levels. With the threshold model (C), maximal risk reduction is achieved at an LDL cholesterol of about 125 mg/dL, with no further reduction at lower LDL levels.

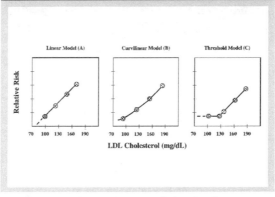

(curvilinear relationship); and the third proposes that a threshold exists below which further lowering of LDL cholesterol produces no additional decrement in risk. Post hoc analysis of the 4S trial supported the curvilinear relationship.[87] In contrast, post hoc analysis of CARE and LIPID trials favored a threshold relationship.[47] According to the latter, further reductions in LDL cholesterol below 125 mg/dL produced no additional decrement in absolute risk for CHD.

It is expected that future clinical trials that specifically address this question will resolve this uncertainty of relationship.

However, the results of the Heart Protection Study (HPS)[16] may have modified the question of the LDL/CHD relationship. The assumptions contained in the above figures suggest that absolute risk for CHD is highly dependent on baseline LDL-cholesterol levels. However, this was not entirely the case in HPS. Although baseline risk was related to LDL cholesterol, even those at low LDL levels remained at relatively high risk. In HPS, statin therapy at fixed dose produced a similar reduction in relative risk, regardless of baseline LDL-cholesterol level. The relationship between changes in LDL-cholesterol levels and CHD risk appeared such as might be called a "rule of thirds." In other words, reduction of LDL cholesterol by one third reduced risk for CHD by one third, regardless of baseline LDL-cholesterol level. Indeed, this "rule of thirds" is supported by all other statin trials.[11-15] If this rule holds, the relationship between LDL-cholesterol levels and CHD risk might be visualized as shown in Figure 8. It hypothesizes that for each successive lowering of LDL cholesterol levels by one-third, the risk for CHD likewise is reduced by one-third regardless of baseline LDL.

According to Figure 8, further risk reduction would be achieved by reducing LDL-cholesterol levels to considerably below 100 mg/dL. Thus the recommendation for "less than 100 mg/dL" could be interpreted as meaning "the lower, the better." Whereas the latter may be true, it may be difficult to reduce LDL-cholesterol to well below 100 mg/dL in many patients. Standard doses of statins will reduce LDL-cholesterol levels by about one-third. These can be recommended in most high-risk patients, regardless of baseline LDL-cholesterol levels. Achieving a reduction of LDL cholesterol by an additional one-third will require either high-dose statins, LDL-cholesterol lowering drugs in combination, or both. For many patients, such aggressive lowering of LDL-cholesterol may not be appropriate on grounds of practicability and safety. For this reason, clinical judgment will be required as to how aggressive to be in LDL lowering in high-risk patients. With current therapies, it will be possible to obtain an additional one-sixth reduction in LDL, beyond the initial one-third, with more aggressive LDL lowering. However, still greater reductions may exceed the bounds of safety with currently available drugs.

Figure 8 - Relation between LDL-cholesterol levels and absolute risk for coronary heart disease in high-risk patients, as suggested by recent data of the Heart Protection Study as well as other statin trials. Although absolute risk is related to baseline LDL-cholesterol levels, even those with a low LDL cholesterol remain at high risk. With LDL-lowering therapy, risk reduction is curvilinear (log-linear). According to the clinical trials, reduction of LDL by one-third reduces risk for CHD by one-third regardless of baseline LDL levels. According to this model, if LDL levels could be lowered by another third, absolute risk for CHD would also be reduced by another one-third.

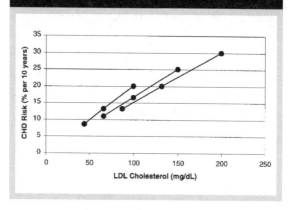

Cost effectiveness of LDL-lowering therapy in high-risk patients. For persons with CHD and CHD risk equivalents, LDL-lowering therapy not only reduces risk for major coronary events and stroke, but it yields highly favorable cost-effectiveness ratios. Cost effectiveness is enhanced by reduction in costs associated with major cardiovascular events.

Recommendations for LDL-lowering therapy according to baseline LDL-cholesterol levels. The following ATP III recommendations pertain to instituting LDL-lowering therapy in patients with CHD and CHD risk equivalents at different baseline levels of LDL cholesterol.

- If baseline LDL cholesterol is ≥130 mg/dL, intensive lifestyle therapy and maximal control of other risk factors should be started immediately. Moreover, for most patients, an LDL-lowering drug will be required to achieve an LDL cholesterol <100 mg/dL; thus an LDL-cholesterol lowering drug can be started simultaneously with TLC to attain the goal of therapy. When LDL-cholesterol levels are <150 mg/dL, standard doses of statins usually will reduce levels to <100 mg/dL. If further reductions are deemed warranted, more aggressive drug therapy will be required. Such will require either higher doses of statins or combining statins with another drug (e.g., bile acid sequestrant or nicotinic acid). If cholesterol-absorption blockers become available, they could be effectively combined with statin therapy. Use of these drugs will make it possible to achieve an additional LDL lowering of approximately 18%. If baseline LDL is

>150 mg/dL, standard doses of statins may not reduce LDL-cholesterol levels to below 100 mg/dL. If not, consideration must be given as to whether to apply more aggressive LDL-lowering therapy.

• If baseline LDL-cholesterol levels are 100-129 mg/dL, several therapeutic approaches are available:

– Initiate or intensify lifestyle and/or drug therapies to lower LDL cholesterol to <100 mg/dL. This is the ATP III preferred approach because it will achieve the goal of therapy for LDL cholesterol in patients with CHD and CHD risk equivalents. This approach also is supported by the recent results of the HPS. At the time of publication of ATP III, the results of the HPS were not available. In light of HPS results, significant risk reduction will be obtained in high-risk patients with statin therapy when baseline LDL-cholesterol levels are in the range of 100-129 mg/dL. A standard dose of statin should reduce LDL-cholesterol levels to the range of 65 to 85 mg/dL. Further LDL lowering probably will not be indicated.

– If on-treatment LDL cholesterol is in the range of 100-129 mg/dL, further LDL lowering will be required to achieve a goal of <100 mg/dL.

Thus, if a patient is already receiving a standard dose of statin, several options are available. A tripling of the statin dose will reduce LDL-cholesterol levels by about 12% more, which will lower LDL-cholesterol levels to the range of 88 to 115 mg/dL. Alternatively, if bile acid sequestrants are added to a standard statin dose, an 18% additional lowering will decrease the LDL-cholesterol level to 80-105 mg/dL, which should be sufficient.

- If serum LDL cholesterol is approaching the optimal level, more emphasis should be given to weight reduction and increased physical activity, especially in persons with the metabolic syndrome. This option does not exclude the benefit of additional LDL lowering, but should enhance risk reduction accompanying LDL-lowering therapy.

- An alternate approach is to institute treatment of other lipid or non-lipid-risk factors. With this option, consideration can be given to use of other lipid-modifying drugs (e.g., nicotinic acid or fibric acid). This option is more attractive if the patient has elevated triglycerides or low HDL cholesterol. One rationale for this approach derives from the VA-HIT trial in which significant risk reduction was achieved by fibrate therapy even when LDL-cholesterol levels were not in the optimal range. Because of HPS, however, priority probably should be given to use of statins even when triglycerides are elevated or HDL-cholesterol levels are reduced. If fibrates or nicotinic acid are to be employed, they likely will be used in combination with statin therapy.

- According to ATP III, if baseline LDL cholesterol is <100 mg/dL, further LDL-lowering therapy is not required. On the other hand, HPS found that initiation of statin therapy significantly reduced risk even when LDL-cholesterol levels were less than 100 mg/dL. The rationale for adding an LDL-lowering drug was presented above. Therefore, the physician has the option to start further LDL lowering in this group of patients. These patients should further still be advised to follow the TLC Diet to help keep the LDL level optimal. Regardless, more emphasis should be placed on controlling other lipid and non-lipid-risk factors and on treatment of the metabolic syndrome, if present.

INTERMEDIATE RISK: MULTIPLE (2+) RISK FACTORS

Many persons are at increased risk for CHD, but their risk is below the high-risk category.

Table 5-Replacement of Framingham Risk Points for Age with Coronary Calcium Scores for Men and Women (Modified from Reference 89)

	Men				Women			
Age	Framingham Age Points	Coronary Calcium Scores			Framingham Age Points	Coronary Calcium Scores		
Years		<25th	25-75th	>75th		<25th	25-75th	>75th
			Percentile				Percentile	
20-34	-9	-12	-9	0	-7	-11	-7	0
35-39	-4	-9	-4	3	-3	-9	-3	3
40-44	0	-6	0	6	0	-6	0	6
45-49	3	-4	3	8	3	-3	3	8
50-54	6	0	6	10	6	0	6	10
55-59	8	3	8	11	8	3	8	12
60-64	10	6	10	12	10	6	10	14
65-69	11	8	11	13	12	8	12	16
70-74	12	10	12	14	14	10	14	18
75-79	13	11	13	15	16	12	16	20

They can be said to have *intermediate risk*. Most patients in this category have multiple (2+) risk factors. ATP III importantly recognizes that there are gradations of risk in the intermediate-risk category. One of the essential features of "primary prevention" in ATP III was the triage of intermediate-risk patients into three groups: (a) some are elevated to the *high-risk* category, (b) others are identified as having *moderately-high risk*, and (c) still others are considered at only *moderate risk*. These distinctions are important because with increasing risk category the intensity of LDL-lowering therapy also is increased. The primary technique used for categorization is Framingham risk scoring. According to this method, major risk factors are weighted and incorporated into Framingham risk equations.

Framingham scoring can be carried out in two ways, either by score sheets or by computer. Table 3 shows scoring sheets for men and women, respectively. Points are entered for the major risk factors: total cholesterol, HDL cholesterol, smoking, blood pressure, and age. Point scores for each risk factor are summed, and 10-year risk for hard CHD (myocardial infarction + coronary death) is obtained. Alternatively, a computer programmed with Framingham risk equations also can be used. Computerized scoring can be obtained from the NHLBI website (www.nhlbi.nih.gov), or the program can be downloaded into a Palm Pilot for risk estimation.

ATP III recommendations for each category of risk in patients with multiple (2+) risk factors can be summarized briefly. Some of these recommendations have been adjusted to employ options of risk assessment implied in ATP III, but not necessarily stated explicitly. Since the publication of ATP III, several advances in risk assessment expand the list of options for classification.

● *Intermediate Risk (2+ Risk Factors)→ High-Risk Status.*

— *Multiple (2+) risk factors and 10-year risk >20%.* When patients with multiple risk factors and apparent intermediate risk have a 10-year risk for hard CHD >20% by Framingham scoring, they can be elevated to the status of CHD risk equivalent. They are managed as described for CHD risk equivalent in the previous section.

Other approaches can be used to identify CHD risk equivalents among patients with multiple risk factors. Although ATP III does not specifically recommend these approaches, it does indicate that they are optional and can be used in selected patients. It must be emphasized however that these alternative approaches are based on a smaller database of information than for Framingham risk scoring. They include the following.

— *Multiple (2+) risk factors and abnormal exercise ECG* in men 45-75 years who have multiple risk factors. Such men apparently have a 10-year risk that appears to exceed 20% and thus can be said to have a CHD risk equivalent.

— *Multiple (2+) risk factors and advanced sub-clinical atherosclerosis.* If a person with multiple risk factors has advanced subclinical atherosclerosis detected either as increased intimal-medial thickness of carotid arteries (detected by B-mode sonography) or increased coronary calcium (detected by electron-beam CT or spiral CT), consideration can be given to elevating the patient to the category of CHD risk equivalent. Two alternate approaches have been proposed for identifying apparently intermediate-risk patients who belong in the category of CHD risk equivalent.

First, Grundy[88,89] has proposed that subclinical atherosclerosis (e.g., coronary calcium) can replace age as a risk factor in Framingham scoring. This proposal is based on the assumption that age is a surrogate marker for coronary plaque burden. If so, coronary calcium scores should provide a better marker for plaque burden than age. Consequently, replacement of age scores with coronary calcium scores should provide an improved prediction of risk. Table 5 provides modified Framingham scoring based on coronary calcium scores.

Second, Greenland et al.[90] suggests that apparently intermediate-risk patients can be elevated to the level of CHD risk equivalent if their subclinical atherosclerosis, whether determined by coronary calcium or carotid IMT, is >75th percentile for age and sex. This technique has the advantage of simplicity, but also may over-recruit persons into the high-risk category. It is not clear that all patients, particularly women, who have 2+ risk factors and ≥75th percentile elevations of subclinical atherosclerosis will have a 10-year risk for CHD >20.

— *Multiple (2+) risk factors + elevated inflammatory markers.* If a person with multiple risk factors also has persistently elevated hs-CRP levels, consideration also can be given to elevation of the person to the high-risk category. A categorical increase in hs-CRP can be taken as levels exceeding the 75th percentile for a reference, healthy population. This value is typically greater than 4 mg/L.[9] This reclassification has the same potential to over-recruit persons into the high risk category, as may occur with the approach of Greenland et al.[90] It must be emphasized however that the evidence-base for raising the risk category of a person with elevated hs-CRP is not as strong as that for advanced subclinical atherosclerosis.

Analysis of costs of LDL-lowering drugs for patients with established CHD has revealed a high level of cost-effectiveness. The literature contains several such analyses, and there is uniform agreement that LDL-lowering drug therapy in CHD patients is highly cost effective.

● *Intermediate Risk (2+ risk factors)*→
 Moderate-to-Moderately High-Risk

For persons with intermediate risk (multiple (2+) risk factors) and 10-year risk for CHD ≤20%, intensity of therapy should be adjusted according to 10-year risk and LDL-cholesterol level. All persons with multiple risk factors and ≤20% risk have a therapeutic goal for LDL cholesterol of <130 mg/dL. This goal was chosen to provide significant benefit from LDL-lowering therapy while at the same time avoiding the excessive costs of drug therapy that would be imposed by the recommendation for a goal of <100 mg/dL in a very large portion of the American public.

— *Multiple (2+) risk factors and a 10-year risk of 10-20%.* In this category, called moderately-high risk, the goal for LDL cholesterol is <130 mg/dL. The therapeutic aim is to reduce short-term risk as well as long-term risk for CHD. If baseline LDL cholesterol is ≥130 mg/dL, therapeutic lifestyle changes are

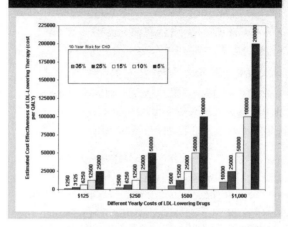

Figure 9—Dependence of cost effectiveness on costs of LDL lowering drugs (modified from ATP III). As 10-year risk for CHD declines, cost per quality adjusted life year (QALY) gained increases. As yearly price of statin therapy decreases, cost per QALY gained declines.

initiated and maintained for 3 months. If LDL remains ≥130 mg/dL after 3 months of the LDL-lowering diet, consideration can be given to starting an LDL-lowering drug to achieve the LDL goal of <130 mg/dL. Use of LDL-lowering drugs at this risk level reduces CHD risk and is cost-effective. Should the LDL fall to less than 130 mg/dL on dietary therapy alone, the latter can be continued without adding drugs.

This guideline represents one of the more innovative recommendations of ATP III. It extends the potential use of LDL-lowering drugs to persons who would not otherwise have been eligible for drug therapy under ATP II. The decision to extend the use of drugs to persons whose LDL-cholesterol levels on dietary therapy are in the range of 130-159 mg/dL was influenced by the benefits observed in participants of the AFCAPS/TexCAPS trial.[14] In this trial, major coronary events were reduced with lovastatin therapy by 30-40% in persons having LDL-cholesterol levels in this range.

In spite of the relative risk reduction with statin therapy in the AFCAPS/TexCAPS study, a portion of the participants had a 10-year risk for hard CHD of <10%. ATP III examined the issue of cost-effectiveness of drug therapy in detail and concluded that at current drug prices, statin therapy is not cost effective when LDL levels are not categorically elevated (≥160 mg/dL) and when 10-year risk is <10%. Drugs are the major factor determining cost-effectiveness of LDL-lowering therapy. The cost effectiveness of drug therapy depends on two major factors: (a) the absolute risk of the patient; and (b) the current costs of drugs. This relationship is shown in Figure 9. This figure reveals that cost per quality adjusted life year (QALY) gained increases as the yearly cost of the drug used in therapy rises. In addition, costs increase as absolute risk declines. According to current standards, an acceptable cost per QALY gained for medical practice ranges from $50,000-100,000 per year or less. As shown in Figure 9, at a cost of $1000 per year, the lower limit of cost effectiveness for statin therapy is an absolute risk for hard CHD of about 10%; at lower levels of risk, costs become prohibitively high. As drug costs decline, nevertheless, drug therapy will be cost effective in lower ranges of absolute risk. Cost effectiveness thus was one factor affecting recommendations about drug therapy in persons with multiple risk factors.

— *Multiple (2+) risk factors and a 10-year risk of <10%.* This category is called *moderate risk.* Here the goal for LDL cholesterol also is <130 mg/dL. The therapeutic aim, however, is primarily to reduce longer-term risk. If baseline LDL cholesterol is ≥130 mg/dL, persons are started on dietary therapy for reducing LDL cholesterol. If LDL is <160 mg/dL on dietary therapy alone, it should be continued without drug intervention. LDL-lowering drugs generally are not recommended because the patient is not at high short-term risk. On the other hand, if LDL cholesterol is ≥160 mg/dL, drug therapy can be considered to achieve an LDL-cholesterol <130 mg/dL; the primary aim is to reduce long-term risk.

In this recommendation, ATP III holds that high long-term risk accompanying high LDL-cholesterol levels (≥160 mg/dL) overrides a marginal cost effectiveness of LDL-lowering drugs. Treatment with drugs in this category of patients can be justified to slow development of coronary atherosclerosis and to reduce long-term risk for CHD. This is not a new recommendation; it was in both ATPs I and II. The recommendation is analogous to the recommendation of the National High Blood Pressure Education Program that categorical hypertension (BP ≥140/90 mmHg) be treated if necessary with drugs. Regarding cost effectiveness, it is expected that over a period of many years there will be a progressive decline in the cost of LDL-lowering drugs. Consequently, cost effectiveness of treatment of elevated LDL cholesterol in this population will improve progressively over time.

- *Magnitude of LDL lowering in primary prevention.* An important question regarding management of LDL cholesterol is how aggressive to be with LDL lowering in primary prevention.

According to current ATP III guidelines, about half of all persons entering clinical management for elevated LDL cholesterol are candidates for dietary therapy without added drugs. Although ATP III emphasizes goals of therapy for persons who enter clinical management of elevated LDL-cholesterol levels, it appears that the investment in clinical therapy calls for substantial LDL lowering to be "cost effective." In accord with the "rule of thirds," discussed before, a general guide might be that if full clinical management is initiated, LDL-cholesterol levels should be reduced by at least one-third to justify the time and expense to physicians and patients. For many patients an LDL reduction of about 30% can be achieved by lifestyle therapies alone. However, others may require the addition of a low dose of drug(s) to achieve such a lowering. Table 6 suggests various modalities that could be employed in a combination of lifestyle and low-dose drug therapy to achieve a one-third reduction in LDL-cholesterol levels. Thus use of low doses of drugs in combination with diet may provide a reasonable approach to the clinical management of elevated LDL cholesterol in primary prevention.[91] This approach should be both safe and cost-effective.

HIGH LIFETIME RISK: INFLUENCE OF SEVERE SINGLE RISK FACTORS

Most persons with 0-1 risk factor have a 10-year risk <10%. Persons with 0-1 risk factors who enter clinical management are those with baseline LDL-cholesterol levels ≥160 mg/dL. The goal for LDL cholesterol in this risk category is a level <160 mg/dL. The primary aim of therapy is to reduce long-term risk. First-line

Table 6–Combination Lifestyle and Low-Dose Drug Therapies for LDL Lowering		
Therapy	Average % Lowering of LDL Cholesterol	Cumulative % Lowering of LDL Cholesterol
Reduced saturated fats and cholesterol in diet	10%	10%
Plant stanol/sterols (2 g/day)	10%	19%
Viscousfi ber (10 g/day)	5%	22%
Weight reduction	5%	26%
Low-dose bile acid sequestrant	15% (8-10g/day)	37%
Very low dose statin (one-fourth standard dose)	15%	48%

therapy is therapeutic lifestyle changes. If after 3 months of dietary therapy LDL cholesterol is <160 mg/dL, dietary therapy is continued.

Some investigators believe that clinical intervention to achieve an LDL-cholesterol level near to optimal (<130 mg/dL) is justified for the whole population. Undoubtedly it would be accompanied by a reduction in relative risk, as shown in the AFCAPS/TexCAPS study.[14] On the other hand, use of LDL-lowering drugs to reduce LDL-cholesterol levels from the range of 130-159 mg/dL to 100-129 mg/dL in otherwise low-risk persons is not cost effective at current drug costs. Further, because of the large number of persons in this category, the absolute costs of drug therapy if widely imposed would be an enormous financial burden on the medical care system.

In contrast, if LDL cholesterol is 160-189 mg/dL after an adequate trial of dietary therapy, drug therapy is optional depending on clinical judgment; factors favoring use of drugs include:

● A severe single risk factor (heavy cigarette smoking, poorly controlled hypertension, strong family history of premature CHD, or very low HDL cholesterol)

- Multiplicity of life-habit risk factors and emerging risk factors (if measured)

- 10-year risk approaching 10% (if measured)

If LDL cholesterol is ≥190 mg/dL in spite of TLC, drug therapy should be considered to achieve the LDL goal of <160 mg/dL.

The purpose of using LDL-lowering drugs in persons with 0-1 risk factor and elevated LDL cholesterol (≥160 mg/dL) is to slow the development of coronary atherosclerosis, which will reduce long-term risk. This aim may conflict with cost-effectiveness considerations; thus clinical judgment is required in selection of persons for drug therapy. Nonetheless, a strong case can be made for using drugs when LDL cholesterol is ≥190 mg/dL after TLC, and for selected persons, when levels range from 160-189 mg/dL.

For persons whose LDL-cholesterol levels are already below the recommended goal upon first encounter, instructions for appropriate changes in life habits, periodic follow-up, and control of other risk factors are needed.

Management of the Metabolic Syndrome: Benefit Beyond Lowering of LDL Cholesterol

In ATP III, priority is given to lowering LDL cholesterol, the primary target of therapy. Clinical trials show that intensive LDL-lowering therapy will reduce risk for major coronary events by 30 to 40%, as well as decreasing the risk for coronary procedures, CHD death, stroke, and total mortality. However, the ideal goal of prevention would be to achieve at least double reduction in risk. To attain this ideal goal, other risk factors must be attacked beyond LDL cholesterol. Risk reduction comparable to that achieved with intensive LDL-lowering therapy can be obtained by cessation of cigarette smoking. Additional risk reduction is possible through modifying the risk factors of the metabolic syndrome. The following outlines approaches to incremental risk reduction through modification of the various components of the metabolic syndrome.

INSULIN RESISTANCE

A major characteristic of patients with the metabolic syndrome is the presence of insulin resistance. Many investigators believe that insulin resistance is a cause of the metabolic risk factors characteristic of this syndrome. Certainly a reduction of insulin resistance will mitigate many of these risk factors. The major causes of insulin resistance are overweight/obesity (especially abdominal obesity), physical inactivity, and genetic factors. The primary and most effective approach to reduction of insulin resistance is weight loss and increased physical activity. For this reason, ATP III places increased emphasis on these lifestyle modifications as a component TLC.

With little doubt, genetic factors predispose some persons to insulin resistance. In such persons, even moderate overweight and physical inactivity can significantly impair insulin sensitivity. There is a growing interest in the possibility that drugs might be used to reduce insulin resistance. Two such agents are metformin and thiazolidinediones (glitazones). At present these agents are largely reserved for reducing insulin resistance in patients with overt diabetes. They are not now recommended for treatment of insulin resistance in patients without diabetes. However, clinical trials are underway to evaluate their efficacy in patients with the metabolic syndrome, and they might be used for this purpose in the future.

ATHEROGENIC DYSLIPIDEMIA

The lipid triad (elevated triglyceride, small LDL particles, and low HDL cholesterol) is common in patients with the metabolic syndrome. Weight reduction and increased physical activity will improve atherogenic dyslipidemia in many persons. In addition, drugs that target atherogenic dyslipidemia have been shown to reduce major coronary events. These include fibric acids and nicotinic acid. Figure 10 shows results of clinical trials with these agents. In all trials there is a trend towards a beneficial effect; and in several of the trials, statistically significant reductions in major coronary events were obtained within the trial itself. On the basis of all the trials, it can be estimated that these drugs will reduce risk for major coronary events by 15-25%.

Figure 10–Risk reduction in major coronary events accompanying drugs that primarily modify Atherogenic Dyslipidemia (modified from ATP III). These drugs include various fibrates and nicotinic acids. In most clinical trials, modification of Atherogenic Dyslipidemia with drug therapy produced a trend towards reduction in CHD risk.

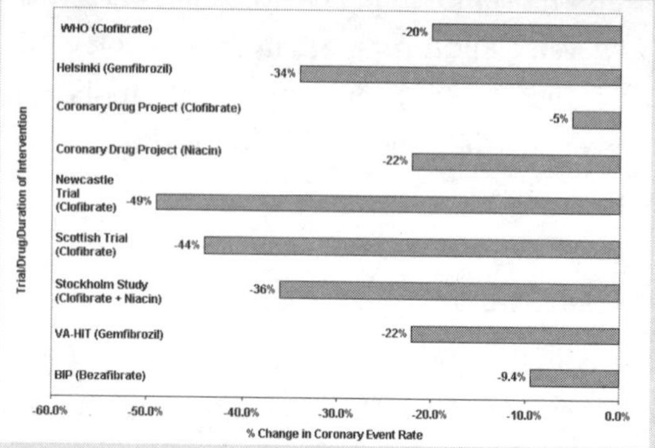

ELEVATED BLOOD PRESSURE

Patients with the metabolic syndrome frequently have elevated blood pressure. In some, the elevation is only to the high normal range (BP = 130-139/85-89 mmHg). In others the blood pressure is raised to that of categorical hypertension (BP ≥140/90 mg/dL). With only moderate elevations in blood pressure, weight reduction and increased physical activity may be sufficient to achieve normal readings. However, those with categorical hypertension may require antihypertensive medications in addition. Treatment of hypertension has been shown to reduce risk for both stroke and major coronary events.

PROTHROMBOTIC STATE

Although the prothrombotic state usually is hidden from view in patients with the metabolic syndrome, a tendency for coronary thrombosis results from increased PAI-1 levels and probably other prothrombotic factors. Low dose aspirin, as shown in both primary and secondary prevention trials, can reduce this tendency for coronary thrombosis. Current recommendations highlight aspirin prophylaxis mainly for secondary prevention, although its use in high-risk patients with the metabolic syndrome may be justifiable. For such patients it is necessary to judiciously balance the benefit in CHD risk reduction with the increased risk for bleeding accompanying aspirin. For example, aspirin therapy in most patients with CHD risk equivalents is justified.

Special Issues
MANAGEMENT OF SPECIFIC DYSLIPIDEMIAS

Very High LDL Cholesterol (>190 mg/dL)

When LDL-cholesterol levels are ≥190 mg/dL, there usually is a genetic component contributing to such high levels. Levels in this range occur in 5-10% of the American population. Monogenic familial hypercholesterolemia occurs in about 1:500 people; familial defective apolipoprotein B has a frequency of about 1:1000. The remaining affected persons have polygenic hypercholesterolemia. Dietary factors generally contribute to very high LDL-cholesterol levels; thus, a 10% reduction in LDL-cholesterol levels with dietary therapy will take many people out of the range of very high LDL. Early detection of high or very high LDL cholesterol in young adults is needed to prevent premature CHD. Family testing is also recommended to identify affected relatives who also have hypercholesterolemia. Most patients with very high LDL levels will require combined drug therapy (e.g., statin + bile acid seques-trant) to achieve the goals of LDL-lowering therapy. Intensive LDL-lowering therapy is par-ticularly necessary for persons with familial hypercholesterolemia to prevent early onset CHD.

Elevated Serum Triglycerides

For many years, elevated serum triglycerides were considered to be unrelated to development of CHD. Recent meta-analyses of prospective studies however indicate that elevated triglyc-erides are an independent risk factor for CHD. Presumably, the independence of prediction is due to high levels of atherogenic lipoproteins associated with high triglycerides. When per-sons are detected with elevated triglycerides, the underlying cause should be sought. Many envi-ronmental factors contribute to higher than nor-mal triglycerides in the general population: obe-sity and overweight, physical inactivity, cigarette smoking, excess alcohol intake, high carbohy-drate diets (>60% of energy intake). Secondary causes of high triglycerides include various dis-eases (e.g., type 2 diabetes, chronic renal failure, nephrotic syndrome), and certain drugs (e.g., corticosteroids, estrogens, retinoids, higher doses of beta-adrenergic blocking agents). Several genetic dyslipidemias are accompanied by elevated triglycerides and premature CHD; most notable are familial combined hyperlipidemia, familial hypertriglyceridemia, and familial dysbetalipoproteinemia.

In clinical practice, elevated serum triglycerides are most often observed in persons with the metabolic syndrome. In the presence of this syndrome, environmental factors (overweight/ obesity and physical inactivity) are dominant causes; nevertheless secondary or genetic factors can heighten triglyceride levels. For example, patients with familial combined hyperlipidemia and familial hypertriglyceridemia often carry the stigmata of the metabolic syndrome.

An innovative feature of ATP III is the introduction of non-HDL cholesterol (VLDL cholesterol + LDL cholesterol) as a secondary target of therapy in persons with hypertriglyceridemia (triglycerides ≥200 mg/dL). In clinical practice, VLDL cholesterol is the most readily available measure of atherogenic remnant lipoproteins. Thus, the sum of VLDL cholesterol and LDL cholesterol can be identified with "atherogenic" cholesterol. The goal for non-HDL cholesterol in persons with high serum triglycerides can be set at 30 mg/dL higher than that for LDL cholesterol on the premise that a VLDL-cholesterol level ≤30 mg/dL is normal. LDL cholesterol remains the primary target of treatment in persons with high triglycerides, but once the LDL goal is attained, attention must be given to achieving the non-HDL cholesterol goal. The following table compares LDL cholesterol and non-HDL cholesterol goals for three risk categories.

Risk Category	LDL-C Goal	Non-HDL-C Goal
CHD and CHD Risk Equivalent (10-year risk for CHD >20%)	<100 mg/dL	<130 mg/dL
Multiple (2+) Risk Factors and 10-year risk ≤20%	<130 mg/dL	<160 mg/dL
0-1 Risk Factor	<160 mg/dL	<190 mg/dL

The treatment strategy for elevated triglycerides depends on the causes of elevation and severity. When triglycerides are borderline high (150-199 mg/dL), they usually signify the presence of the metabolic syndrome; emphasis thus should be placed on weight reduction and increased physical activity. For high triglycerides (200-500 mg/dL), non-HDL cholesterol becomes a secondary target of therapy. Besides weight reduction and increased physical activity, drug therapy can be considered in high-risk persons to achieve the non-HDL cholesterol goal. Two alternative approaches to drug therapy exist. Both require prior attainment of the LDL-cholesterol goal. First, the non-HDL-cholesterol goal can be reached by intensifying therapy with an LDL-lowering drug; but alternatively, nicotinic acid or fibrate can be added to achieve the non-HDL cholesterol goal by further reducing VLDL cholesterol. In rare persons in whom triglycerides are very high (>500 mg/dL), the initial aim of therapy is to prevent acute pancreatitis through triglyceride lowering. This approach requires very low fat diets (≤15% of calorie intake), weight reduction, increased physical activity, and usually a triglyceride-lowering drug (fibrate or nicotinic acid). Only after triglyceride levels have been lowered to <500 mg/dL should attention turn to LDL lowering to reduce risk for CHD.

Low HDL Cholesterol

Low HDL cholesterol is a strong independent predictor of CHD. In ATP III, low HDL cholesterol is defined categorically as a level <40 mg/dL, a change from the level of <35 mg/dL in ATP II. In the present guidelines, low HDL cholesterol both modifies the goal for LDL-lowering therapy and is used as a risk factor to estimate 10-year risk for CHD. The higher cutpoint for categorically low HDL cholesterol in ATP III was based on evidence that moderately low levels of HDL often signify the presence of the metabolic syndrome. They call for more clinical attention to the need for introducing therapeutic lifestyle changes. Moreover, in clinical trials, the greatest absolute benefit of LDL-lowering therapy was observed in subgroups whose HDL-cholesterol levels were below 40 mg/dL.

ATP III does not specify a goal for HDL raising, e.g., a level ≥40 mg/dL. Although clinical trial results suggest that raising HDL will reduce risk, the evidence is insufficient to specify a target goal for HDL-raising therapy. Unfortunately, currently available drugs other than nicotinic acid do not robustly raise HDL cholesterol, and this drug is often accompanied by side effects. Until improved HDL-raising drugs become available, it will be difficult to test the efficacy of such an approach in large clinical trials. Nonetheless, a low HDL level should receive clinical attention. LDL lowering takes precedence over HDL raising even in persons with low HDL. Moreover, after the LDL goal has been reached, the metabolic syndrome becomes the next target of treatment; for its management, weight reduction and increased physical activity constitute the preferred approach. ATP III concludes that therapeutic lifestyle changes have more to offer most people with low HDL levels than drug therapy that specifically targets HDL. Furthermore, when a low HDL cholesterol occurs in the presence of high triglycerides (200-500 mg/dL), non-HDL cholesterol becomes the secondary target of therapy. Treatment of low HDL cholesterol with drugs in primary prevention is open to the issue of unproven long-term benefit of HDL raising. On the other hand, in the presence of CHD or CHD risk equivalents, a more aggressive approach to low HDL can be taken. For example, drugs that raise HDL (e.g., fibrates or nicotinic acid) deserve consideration when LDL levels are near optimal levels and HDL levels remain low.

Diabetic Dyslipidemia

Diabetic dyslipidemia essentially represents atherogenic dyslipidemia occurring in persons with type 2 diabetes. Elevated triglycerides and/or low HDL cholesterol have long been thought to be the major lipid disorder in patients with type 2 diabetes. Still, the risk reduction in recent clinical trials with statin therapy, when used for patients with diabetes support the identification of LDL-cholesterol as the primary target of treatment. Although drugs that lower triglycerides or raise HDL may be beneficial in patients with diabetes, their usage does not have the strong evidence base that exists for LDL-lowering therapy. Moreover, since diabetes is designated a CHD risk equivalent in ATP III, the LDL-cholesterol goal of therapy for most patients with diabetes is <100 mg/dL. The rationale for LDL management for patients with diabetes is similar to that for CHD patients. When LDL cholesterol is ≥130 mg/dL, most persons with diabetes (both type 1 and type 2) will require initiation of LDL-lowering drugs simultaneously with therapeutic lifestyle changes to achieve the LDL goal. When LDL-cholesterol levels are in the range of 100-129 mg/dL at baseline or on treatment, several therapeutic options are available: increasing intensity of LDL-lowering therapy, adding a drug to modify atherogenic dyslipidemia (fibrate or nicotinic acid), or intensifying control of other risk factors including hyperglycemia. When triglyceride levels are ≥200 mg/dL, non-HDL cholesterol becomes a secondary target of cholesterol-lowering therapy.

SPECIAL CONSIDERATIONS FOR DIFFERENT POPULATION GROUPS

Middle-aged Men (35-65 Years)

In general, men have a higher risk for CHD than

do women. Middle-aged men in particular have a high prevalence of the major risk factors and are predisposed to abdominal obesity and the metabolic syndrome. A sizable fraction of all CHD in men occurs in middle age. Thus, many middle-aged men carry a relatively high risk for CHD, and for those who do, intensive LDL-lowering therapy is needed. Since CHD is common in middle-aged men, most controlled clinical trials of cholesterol-lowering therapy have been carried out predominantly in this population. The results of benefit obtained in recent clinical trials are robust. The increasing population of this age group (i.e., "baby boomers") accounts in part for the expanding need for cholesterol-lowering drugs in the United States.

Women (Ages 45-75 Years)

The onset of CHD in women generally is delayed by some 10-15 years compared to men; for this reason, most CHD in women occurs after age 65. Nevertheless a significant minority of women are at risk for premature CHD. All risk factors contribute to CHD in women, and most premature CHD in women (<65 years) occurs in those with multiple risk factors and the metabolic syndrome. It should be noted that the prevalence of type 2 diabetes, which is a CHD risk equivalent, is just as high in women as in men. This finding implies a high prevalence of the metabolic syndrome in women and reveals a portion of the population who are at higher risk.

In spite of the previous belief that the gender difference in risk for CHD reflects a protective effect of estrogen in women, recent secondary and primary prevention trials cast doubt on the use of hormone-replacement therapy to reduce CHD risk in postmenopausal women. In contrast, the favorable effects of statin therapy in women in clinical trials make a cholesterol-lowering drug preferable to hormone-replacement therapy for CHD risk reduction. Certainly for secondary pre-vention women should be treated similarly to men, i.e., frequent use of LDL-lowering drugs. For primary prevention, ATP III's general approach is similarly applicable for women and men. However, the later onset of CHD for women in general should be factored into clinical decisions about use of cholesterol-lowering drugs. Nonetheless, in the final analysis, just as many women die from CHD as do men. Thus, serious attention must be given to both prevention and treatment of CHD in women.

Older Adults (Men ≥65 Years and Women ≥75 Years)

Overall, most new CHD events and most coro-nary deaths occur in older persons (≥65 years).

Secondary prevention trials with statins have included a sizable number of older persons, mostly in the age range of 65 to 75 years. In these trials, older persons showed significant risk reduction with statin therapy. Therefore, older persons with CHD should not be denied the benefit of LDL-lowering therapy simply on the basis of age. On the other hand, clinical judgment is always required for making clinical decisions in older persons who often have complex medical problems.

High LDL cholesterol and low HDL cholesterol still carry predictive power for the development of new-onset CHD in older persons. For primary prevention, therapeutic lifestyle changes are the first line of therapy for older persons. It must be noted however that LDL-cholesterol levels lose some of their predictive power in persons of advancing age. Consideration therefore might be given to adding measures of subclinical atherosclerosis to risk assessment in older persons for the purpose of primary prevention. Those persons with a heavy coronary plaque burden can be given priority in the aggressive reduction of risk factors.

Younger Adults (Men 20-35 Years; Women 20-45 Years)

CHD is rare in these age groups except in those with severe risk factors, e.g., familial hypercholesterolemia, heavy cigarette smoking, or diabetes. Even though the onset of CHD is relatively rare in young adults, coronary atherosclerosis in its early stages may still progress rapidly. Recent studies show that the rate of development of coronary atherosclerosis earlier in life correlates with the major risk factors. In particular, long-term prospective studies reveal that elevated serum cholesterol detected in young adulthood predicts a higher rate of premature CHD in middle age. Thus, risk factor identification in young adults is an important aim for long-term prevention. The combination of early detection and early intervention to control elevated LDL cholesterol with life-habit changes offers the opportunity for delaying or preventing onset of CHD later in life. For young adults with LDL-cholesterol levels ≥130 mg/dL, therapeutic lifestyle changes should be instituted and emphasized. Particular attention should be given to young men who smoke and have a high LDL cholesterol (160-189 mg/dL); they may be candidates for LDL-lowering drugs. When young adults have very high LDL-cholesterol levels (≥190 mg/dL), drug therapy should be considered, as in other adults. Those with severe genetic forms of hypercholesterolemia may

require LDL-lowering drugs in combination
(e.g., statin + bile acid sequestrant).

With these recommendations, ATP III
departs somewhat from those in other countries
that favor first testing of cholesterol at age 35 or
higher. The argument has been made that there
is no "proof" that early intervention will prevent CHD later in life. ATP reports have consis-
tently disagreed with the recommendation for
not testing until later in life. Although it is
impossible to carry out a lifetime prospective
study of cholesterol-lowering therapy, epidemiological and pathology studies demonstrate
unequivocally that atherosclerosis begins in adolescence or early adulthood and is accelerated by
the presence of risk factors. Ultimately, total
coronary plaque burden becomes the over-riding
risk factor for development of CHD. Thus
efforts to prevent atherogenesis beginning early
in life offer the best opportunity for reducing the
high prevalence of CHD in our society.

Racial and Ethnic Groups

African Americans have the highest overall CHD
mortality rate and the highest out-of-hospital
coronary death rates of any ethnic group in the
United States, particularly at younger ages.
Although the reasons for the excess CHD mortality among African Americans have not been

fully determined, it can be accounted for, at least in part, by the high prevalence of coronary risk factors. Hypertension, left ventricular hypertrophy, diabetes mellitus, cigarette smoking, obesity, physical inactivity, and multiple CHD risk factors all occur more frequently in African Americans than in Caucasians. In the NHLBI workshop on validation of Framingham risk scoring, the Framingham risk algorithm was found to predict CHD well in African Americans. The only exception was that hypertension carries a greater relative risk for cardiovascular mortality in African Americans that in white Americans. This relationship thus might be kept in mind when applying Framingham scoring to African Americans. On the other hand, it is not certain whether the higher cardiovascular mortality accompanying hypertension in African Americans can be overcome by more aggressive cholesterol-lowering therapy.

Other ethnic groups and minority populations in the United States include Hispanics, Native Americans, Asian and Pacific Islanders, and South Asians. Although limited data suggest that racial and ethnic groups vary somewhat in baseline risk for CHD, this evidence did not appear sufficient to lead the ATP III panel to modify general recommendations for cholesterol management in these populations.

Adherence to LDL-Lowering Therapy

Adherence to the ATP III guidelines by both patients and providers is a key to approximating the magnitude of the benefits demonstrated in clinical trials of cholesterol lowering. Adherence issues have to be addressed in order to attain the highest possible levels of CHD risk reduction. Thus, ATP III recommends the use of state-of-the-art multidisciplinary methods targeting the patient, providers, and health delivery systems to achieve the full population effectiveness of the guidelines for primary and secondary prevention.

REFERENCES

1. Expert Panel on Detection Evaluation, and Treatment of High Blood Cholesterol in Adults: Executive summary of the third report of the National Cholesterol Education Program (NCEP) expert panel on detection, evaluation, and treatment of high blood cholesterol in adults (Adult Treatment Panel III). *JAMA* 2001;285:2508-2509.

2. The 1988 report of the joint national committee on detection, evaluation, and treatment of high blood pressure. *Arch Int Med* 1988;148:1023-1038.

3. Lipid Research Clinics Program: The Lipid Research Clinics coronary primary prevention trial results: I. Reduction in the incidence of coronary heart disease. *JAMA* 1984;251:351-364.

4. Expert Panel on Detection Evaluation, and Treatment of High Blood Cholesterol in Adults: National Cholesterol Education Program: second report of the Expert Panel on Detection, Evaluation, and Treatment of high blood

cholesterol (Adult Treatment Panel II). *Circulation* 1994;89:1333-1445.

5. Lee TH, Cleeman JI, Grundy SM, et al.: Clinical goals and performance measures for cholesterol management in secondary prevention of coronary heart disease. *JAMA* 2000;283:94-98.

6. *Cholesterol-Lowering Therapy: Evaluation of Clinical Trial Evidence,* New York City, Marcel Dekker, Inc., 2000.

7. Holmes CL, Schulzer M, Mancini GBJ: Angiographic results of lipid-lowering trials: a systematic review and meta-analysis, in Grundy SM (ed): *Cholesterol-Lowering Therapy: Evaluation of Clinical Trial Evidence.* New York City, Marcel Dekker, Inc., 2000, pp 191-220.

8. Navab M, Berliner JA, Watson AD, et al.: The yin and yang of oxidation in the development of the fatty streak. *Arterioscler Thromb Vasc Biol* 1996;16:831-842.

9. Libby P, Ridker PM, Maseri A: Inflammation and atherosclerosis. *Circulation* 2002;105:1135-1143.

10. Gordon DJ: Cholesterol lowering reduces total mortality: the statins, in Grundy SM (ed): *Cholesterol-Lowering Therapy: Evaluation of Clinical Trial Evidence.* New York City, Marcel Dekker, Inc., 2000, pp 299-311.

11. Scandinavian Simvastatin Survival Study Group: Randomised trial of cholesterol lowering in 4444 patients with coronary heart disease: the Scandinavian Simvastatin Survival Study (4S). *Lancet* 1994;344:1383-1389.

12. Sacks FM, Pfeffer MA, Moye LA, et al: The effect of pravastatin on coronary events after myocardial infarction in patients with average cholesterol levels. *N Engl J Med* 1996;335:1001-1009.

13. The Long-Term Intervention with Pravastatin in Ischaemic Disease (LIPID) Study Group: Prevention of cardiovascular events and death with pravastatin in patients with coronary heart disease and a broad range of initial cholesterol levels. *N Engl J Med* 1998;339: 1349-1357.

14. Shepherd J, Cobbe SM, Ford I, et al: Prevention of coronary heart disease with pravastatin in men with hypercholesterolemia. West of Scotland Coronary Prevention Study Group. *N Engl J Med* 1995;333:1301-1307.

15. Downs JR, Clearfield M, Whitney E, Shapiro D, Beere PA, Gotto AM: Primary prevention of acute coronary events with lovastatin in men and women with average cholesterol levels. Results of AFCAPS/TexCAPS. *JAMA* 1998;279:1615-1622.

16. Heart Protection Study Collaborative Group. MRC/BHF Heart Protection Study of cholesterol lowering with simvastatin in 20,536 high-risk individuals: a randomized placebo-controlled trial. *The Lancet* 2002;360:7-22.

17. Law MR, Wald NJ, Thompson SG: By how much and how quickly does reduction in serum cholesterol concentration lower risk of ischaemic heart disease? *Br Med J* 1994;308:367-372.

18. McGill HC Jr, McMahan CA, Herderick EE, et al.: Effects of coronary heart disease risk factors on atherosclerosis of selected regions of the aorta and right coronary artery. PDAY research group. Pathobiological Determinants of Atherosclerosis in Youth. *Arterioscler Thromb Vasc Biol* 2000;20:836-845.

19. Davies MJ: Going from immutable to mutable atherosclerotic plaques. *Am J Cardiol* 2001;88 (4 Suppl):2F-9F.

20. Libby P: Current concepts of the pathogenesis of the acute coronary syndromes. *Circulation* 2001;104:365-372.

21. Grundy SM, D'Agostino RB, Mosca L, et al.: Cardiovascular risk assessment based on US cohort studies: findings from a National Heart Lung and Blood Institute Workshop. *Circulation* 2001;104:491-496.

22. D'Agostino RB Sr, Grundy S, Sullivan LM, Wilson P, CHD Risk Prediction Group: Validation of the Framingham coronary heart disease prediction scores: results of a multiple ethnic groups investigation. *JAMA* 2001;286:180-187.

23. Smith SC Jr, Greenland P, Grundy SM: AHA Conference Proceedings. Prevention Conference V: Beyond secondary prevention: Identifying the high-risk patient for primary prevention: executive summary. American Heart Association. *Circulation* 2000;101:111-116.

24. National Institutes of Health: Clinical guidelines on the identification, evaluation, and treatment of overweight and obesity in adults—the evidence report. *Obes Res* 1998;2:51S-209S.

25. Festa A, D'Agostino R Jr, Williams K, et al.: The relation of body fat mass and distribution to markers of chronic inflammation. *Int J Obes Relat Metab Disord* 2001;25:1407-1415.

26. Tchernof A, Nolan A, Sites CK, Ades PA, Poehlman ET: Weight loss reduces C-reactive protein levels in obese postmenopausal women. *Circulation* 2002;10:564-569.

27. Mavri A, Alessi MC, Bastelica D, et al.: Subcutaneous abdominal, but not femoral fat expression of plasminogen activator inhibitor-1 (PAI-1) is related to plasma PAI-1 levels and insulin-resistance and decreases after weight loss. *Diabetologia* 2001;44:2025-2031.

28. Mertens I, Van der Planken M, Corthouts B, et al.: Visceral fat is a determinant of PAI-1 activity in diabetic and non-diabetic overweight and obese women. *Horm Metab Res* 2001;33:602-607.

29. Mayer-Davis EJ, D'Agostino R Jr, Karter AJ, et al.: Intensity and amount of physical activity in relation to insulin sensitivity: the Insulin Resistance Atherosclerosis Study. *JAMA* 1998;279:669-674.

30. Assanelli B, Bersatti F, Ferrari R, et al.: Effect of leisure time and working activity on principal risk factors and relative interactions in active middle-aged men. *Coronary Artery Dis* 1999;10:1-7.

31. Liese AD, Mayer-Davis EJ, Tyroler HA, et al.: Development of the multiple metabolic syndrome in the ARIC cohort: joint contribution of insulin, BMI, and WHR. Atherosclerosis risk in communities. *Ann Epidemiol* 1997;7:407-416.

32. Gray RS, Fabsitz RR, Cowan LD, Lee ET, Howard BV, Savage PJ: Risk factor clustering in the insulin resistance syndrome. The Strong Heart Study. *Am J Epidemiol* 1998;148:869-878.

33. McKeigue PM, Ferrie JE, Pierpoint T, Marmot MG: Association of early-onset coronary heart disease in South Asian men with glucose intolerance and by hyper-insulinemia. *Circulation* 1993;87(1):152-161.

34. Chandalia M, Abate N, Garg A, Stray-Gundersen J, Grundy SM: Relationship between generalized and upper body obesity to insulin resistance in Asian Indian men. *J Clin Endocrinol Metab* 1999;84:2329-2335.

35. Miller GJ, Beckles GL, Maude GH, et al.: Ethnicity and other characteristics predictive of coronary heart disease in a developing community: principal results of the St. James Survey, Trinidad. *Int J Epidemiol* 1989;18:808-817.

36. Chan JC, Ng MC, Critchley JA, Lee SC, Cockram CS: Diabetes mellitus—a special medical challenge from a Chinese perspective. *Diabetes Res Clin Pract* 2001;54 Suppl 1:S19-S27.

37. Lee J, Heng D, Chia KS, Chew SK, Tan BY, Hughes K: Risk factors and incident coronary heart disease in Chinese, Malay and Asian Indian males: the Singapore Cardiovascular Cohort Study. *Int J Epidemiol* 2001;30:983-988.

38. Mahley RW, Palaoglu KE, Atak Z, et al.: The Turkish Heart Study: lipids, lipoproteins, and apolipoproteins. *J Lipid Res* 1995;36:839-859.

39. Pugeat M, Ducluzeau PH, Mallion-Donadieu M: Association of insulin resistance with hyperandrogenia in women. *Horm Res* 2000;54:322-326.

40. Grundy SM: The optimal ratio of fat-to-carbohydrate in the diet. *Annu Rev Nutr* 1999;19:325-341.

41. Muller DC, Elahi D, Tobin JD, Andres R: The effect of age on insulin resistance and secretion: a review. *Semin Nephrol* 1996;16:289-298.

42. Ford ES, Giles WH, Dietz WH: Prevalence of the metabolic syndrome among US adults. Findings from the Third National Health and Nutrition Survey. *JAMA* 2002;287:356-359.

43. U.S.Department of Health and Human Services: *Physical Activity and Health: A Report of the Surgeon General,* Atlanta, Georgia, US Dept Health Human Services; Centers for Disease Control and Prevention; Natl Center for Chronic Disease Prevention and Health Promotion, 1996.

44. Grundy SM: HMG-CoA reductase inhibitors for treatment of hypercholesterolemia. *N Engl J Med* 1988;319:24-33.

45. Endo A: The discovery and development of HMG CoA reductase inhibitors. *J Lipid Res* 1992;33:1569-1582.

46. Staffa JA, Chang J, Green L: Cerivastatin and reports of fatal rhabdomyolysis. *N Engl J Med* 2002;346:539-540.

47. Sacks FM, Moye LA, Davis BR, et al.: Relationship between plasma LDL concentrations during treatment with pravastatin and recurrent coronary events in the Cholesterol and Recurrent Events trial. *Circulation* 1998;97:1446-1452.

48. Goldberg RB, Mellies MJ, Sacks FM, et al.: Cardiovascular events and their reduction with pravastatin in diabetic and glucose-intolerant myocardial infarction survivors with average cholesterol levels. Subgroup analyses in the Cholesterol and Recurrent Events (CARE) Trial. *Circulation* 1998;98:2513-2519.

49. Sacks FM, Tonkin AM, Craven T, et al.: Coronary heart disease in patients with low LDL-cholesterol: benefit of pravastatin in diabetics and enhanced role for HDL-cholesterol and triglycerides as risk factors. *Circulation* 2002;105:1424-1428.

50. Bilheimer DW, Grundy SM, Brown MS, Goldstein JL: Mevinolin and colestipol stimulate receptor-mediated clearance of low density lipoprotein from plasma in familial hypercholesterolemia heterozygotes. *Proc Natl Acad Sci USA* 1983;80:4124-4128.

51. Grundy SM, Vega GL, Bilheimer DW: Influence of combined therapy with mevinolin and interruption of bile-acid reabsorption on low density lipoproteins in heterozygous familial hypercholesterolemia. *Ann Intern Med* 1985;103:339-343.

52. Vega GL, Grundy SM: Treatment of primary moderate hypercholesterolemia with lovastatin (mevinolin) and colestipol. *JAMA* 1987;257:33-38.

53. Garg A, Grundy SM: Cholestyramine therapy for dyslipidemia in non-insulin-dependent diabetes mellitus: a short-term, double-blind, crossover trial. *Ann Intern Med* 1994;121:416-422.

54. Insull W Jr, Toth P, Mullican W, et al.: Effectiveness of colesevelam hydrochloride in decreasing LDL cholesterol in patients with primary hypercholesterolemia: a 24-week randomized controlled trial. *Mayo Clin Proc* 2001;76:971-982.

55. Hunninghake D, Insull W Jr, Toth P, Davidson D, Donovan JM, Burke SK: Coadministration of colesevelam hydrochloride with atorvastatin lowers LDL cholesterol additively. *Atherosclerosis* 2001;158:407-416.

56. Knapp HH, Schrott H, Ma P, et al.: Efficacy and safety of combination simvastatin and colesevelam in patients with primary hypercholesterolemia. *Am J Med* 2001;110:352-360.

57. Miettinen TA, Puska P, Gylling H, Vanhanen H, Vartiainen E: Reduction of serum cholesterol with sitostanol-ester margarine in a mildly hypercholesterolemic population. *N Engl J Med* 1995;333:1308-1312.

58. Plat J, van Onselen EN, van Heugten MM, Mensink RP: Effects on serum lipids, lipoproteins and fat soluble antioxidant concentrations of consumption frequency of margarines and shortenings enriched with plant stanol esters. *Eur J Clin Nutr* 2000;54:671-677.

59. Blair SN, Capuzzi DM, Gottlieb SO, Nguyen T, Morgan JM, Cater NB: Incremental reduction of serum total cholesterol and low-density lipoprotein cholesterol with

the addition of plant stanol ester-containing spread to statin therapy. *Am J Cardiol* 2000;86:46-52.

60. Law M: Plant Sterol and stanol margarines and health. *Br Med J* 2000;320:861-864.

61. Cater NB: Plant stanol ester: review of cholesterol-lowering efficacy and implications for coronary heart disease risk reduction. *Prev Cardiol* 2000;3:121-130.

62. Ezzet F, Wexler D, Statkevich P, et al.: The plasma concentration and LDL-C relationship in patients receiving ezetimibe. *Clin Pharmacol* 2001;41:943-949.

63. Bays HE, Moore PB, Drehobl MA, et al.: Effectiveness and toleratiblity of ezetimibe in patients with primary hypercholesterolemia: pooled analysis of two phase II studies. *Clin Ther* 2001;23:1209-1230.

64. Coronary Drug Project Research Group: Clofibrate and niacin in coronary heart disease. *JAMA* 1975;231:360-381.

65. Carlson LA, Rosenhamer G: Reduction of mortality in the Stockholm ischemic heart disease secondary prevention study to combined treatment with clofibrate and nicotinic acid. *Acta Med Scand* 1988;223:405-418.

66. Canner PL, Berge KG, Wenger NK, for the Coronary Drug Project Research Group: Fifteen year mortality in coronary drug project patients: long-term benefit with niacin. *J Am Coll Cardiol* 1986;8:1245-1255.

67. Gibbons LW, Gonzalez V, Gordon N, Grundy SM: The prevalence of side effects with regular and sustained-release nicotinic acid. *Am J Med* 1995;99:378-385.

68. Vega GL, Grundy SM: Lipoprotein responses to treatment with lovastatin, gemfibrozil, and nicotinic acid in normolipidemic patients with hypoalphalipoproteinemia. *Arch Intern Med* 1994;154:73-82.

69. Guyton JR, Blazing MA, Hagar J, et al.: Extended-release niacin vs gemfibrozil for the treatment of low levels of high-density lipoprotein cholesterol. Niaspan-Gemfibrozil Study Group. *Arch Intern Med* 2000;160:1177-1184.

70. Goldberg A, Alagona P Jr, Capuzzi DM, et al.: Multiple-dose efficacy and safety of an extended-release form of niacin in the management of hyperlipidemia. *Am J Cardiol* 2000;85:1100-1105.

71. Kashyap ML, McGovern ME, Berra K, et al.: Long-term safety and efficacy of a once-daily niacin/lovastatin formulation for patients with dyslipidemia. *Am J Cardiol* 2002;89:672-678.

72. Garg A, Grundy SM: Nicotinic acid as therapy for dyslipidemia in non-insulin-dependent diabetes mellitus. *JAMA* 1990;264:723-726.

73. Elam MB, Hunninghake DB, Davis KB, et al.: Effect of niacin on lipid and lipoprotein levels and glycemic control in patients with diabetes and peripheral arterial disease: the ADMIT study: A randomized trial. Arterial Disease Multiple Intervention Trial. *JAMA* 2000;284:1263-1270.

74. Grundy SM, Vega GL, McGovern M, et al.: Efficacy, safety, and tolerability of once-daily niacin for the treatment of dyslipidemia associated with type 2 diabetes: Results of the Assessment of Diabetes Control and Evaluation of the Efficacy of Niaspan Trial (ADVENT). *Arch Int Med* 2002 (in press).

75. Brown G, Albers JJ, Fisher LD, et al.: Regression of coronary artery disease as a result of intensive lipid-lowering therapy in men with high levels of apolipoprotein B. *N Engl J Med* 1990;323:1289-1298.

76. Brown BG, Zhao XQ, Chait A, et al.: Simvastatin and niacin, antioxidant vitamins, or the combination for the prevention of coronary disease. *N Engl J Med* 2001;345:1583-1592.

77. Fruchart JC, Duriez P, Staels B: Peroxisome proliferator-activated receptor-alpha activators regulate genes governing lipoprotein metabolism, vascular inflammation and atherosclerosis. *Curr Opin Lipidol* 1999;10:245-257.

78. Fruchart JC: Peroxisome proliferator-activated receptor-alpha activation and high-density lipoprotein metabolism. *Am J Cardiol* 2001;88 (12A):24N-29N.

79. Report from the Committee of Principal Investigators: WHO cooperative trial on primary prevention of ischaemic heart disease with clofibrate to lower serum cholesterol: final mortality follow-up. *Lancet* 1984;2:600-604.

80. Frick MH, Elo O, Haapa K, et al.: Helsinki Heart Study: primary prevention trial with gemfibrozil in middle-aged men with dyslipidemia: safety of treatment, changes in risk factors, and incidence of coronary heart disease. *N Engl J Med* 1987;317:1237-1245.

81. Secondary prevention by raising HDL cholesterol and reducing triglycerides in patients with coronary artery disease: the Bezafibrate Infarction Prevention (BIP) study. *Circulation* 2000;102:21-27.

82. Rubins HB, Robins SJ, Collins D, et al.: Gemfibrozil for the secondary prevention of coronary heart disease in men with low levels of high-density lipoprotein cholesterol. Veterans Affairs High-Density Lipoprotein Cholesterol Intervention Trial Study Group. *N Engl J Med* 1999;341:410-418.

83. de Faire U, Ericsson CG, Grip L, Nilsson J, Svane B, Hamsten A: Secondary preventive potential of lipid-lowering drugs. The Bezafibrate Coronray Atherosclerosis Intervention Trial (BECAIT). *Eur Heart J* 1996;17 (Suppl F):37-42.

84. Frick MH, Syvanne M, Nieminen MS, Kauma H, Taskinen MR, for the Lipid Coronary Angiography Trial (LOCAT) Study Group: Prevention of the angiographic progression of coronary and vein-graft atherosclerosis by gemfibrozil after coronary bypass surgery in men with low levels of HDL cholesterol. *Circulation* 1997;96:2137-2143.

85. Effect of fenofibrate on progression of coronary-artery disease in type 2 diabetes: the Diabetes Atherosclerosis Intervention Study, a randomised study. *Lancet* 2001;357:905-910.

86. Grundy SM: Statin trials and goals of cholesterol-lowering therapy. *Circulation* 1998;97:1436-1439.

87. Pedersen TR, Olsson AG, Faergeman O, et al.: Lipoprotein changes and reduction in the incidence of major coronary heart disease events in the Scandinavian Simvastatin Survival Study (4S). *Circulation* 1998;97:1453-1460.

88. Grundy SM: Age as a risk factor: you are as old as your arteries. *Am J Cardiol* 1999;83:1455-1457.

89. Grundy SM: Coronary plaque as a replacement for age as a risk factor in global risk assessment. *Am J Cardiol* 2001;88(2-A):8E-11E.

90. Greenland P, Smith SC Jr, Grundy SM: Improving coronary heart disease risk assessment in asymptomatic people: role of traditional risk factors and noninvasive cardiovascular tests. *Circulation* 2001;104:1863-1867.

91. Denke MA, Grundy SM: Efficacy of low-dose cholesterol lowering drug therapy in men with moderate hypercholesterolemia. *Arch Intern Med* 1995;155:393-399.

Index

R